INTRO FROM
CODY ZULFER

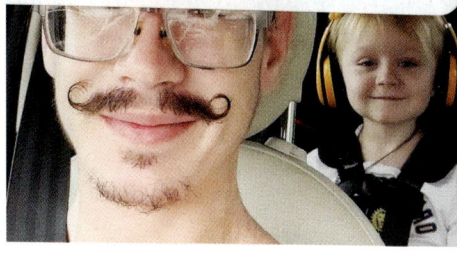

My name is Cody Zulfer.

I'm just a regular Florida guy who loves food. I have suffered from epilepsy since my highschool years. I have a background in competitive surfing and have also been a competitive Brazilian Jiu-jitsu practitioner for the better part of a decade.

About my epilepsy, from high school until my son was about two years old, I was having almost daily seizures. Some days I would have multiple. Doctors were never able to pinpoint the root cause. I was also what they called "a non-responder to medications" leaving every day a gamble of life.

After my son was born, I pushed my Jiu-jitsu training to the side and focused on raising him. Unfortunately, I quickly found my diet going downhill. I was gaining weight and a host of issues came along with that: arthritis, digestive issues, depression, and my energy levels tanked.

The worse my diet got, the worse my seizures became and I didn't understand the correlation. Neither did any doctor I had gone to.

All of this was happening as my son was growing into a very active toddler. He wanted to run and play all the time, but sadly I didn't have the energy. I truly felt I had lost the ability to play with him because my body hurt all the time and I had zero drive. I needed to change!

I started off with fasting. Then moved into keto quickly after. Keto bridged the ignorance gap by bringing my seizures to a halt. I also dropped around 30 pounds in nine months, but some problematic issues remained. A majority of which were digestion-related.

Around that time I began hearing more and more about the carnivore diet. It had sparked hours of self-research. I learned about the complications plant toxins and anti-nutrients have on the body. Contrasting with how rich in vitamins and other beneficial nutrients animal-based proteins and fats really are. I was ready to jump in!

The Ultimate Carnivore Cookbook
www.bioptimizedketo.com

Instagram: GoatFit_Nutrition
Facebook: cody.zulfer

INTRO FOR CODY ZULFER

Once I had given it a try, I was hooked. Within three months I had dropped another 50 pounds. I'd gone from 15% body fat down to 10% and I was putting on lean muscle at the same time. My digestive issues had disappeared, my depression faded away, and I felt great!

As for my son, I had gradually taken out the majority of socially accepted food and snacks an average kid is expected to have. Being an epileptic, I was concerned he could develop it as well. It only made sense that if *this way of eating* had saved me from potential life-threatening seizures, it would save him from ever having to experience it.

I wanted my son as close to meat-based as possible, but I also wanted him to have fun, and enjoy his food. Not that steak isn't fun, but I wanted him to enjoy the same things other kids get to experience: pizza, corn dogs, cheeseburger, etc.

That's really when I got to thinking, "How can I create food the average person would consume regularly, but make them carnivore-based?" Whether it's zero carbs or very low-carb, I really wanted to create forms of the "standard American style food" people love but make them healthy and beneficial to consume.

I love every moment with my son. He drove me to change. Everything I did was for him because I wanted to be a better dad. I didn't want to be this fat guy sitting on the couch, like a giant shadow of the guy I used to be. I wanted to be the best I could be... FOR HIM.

As far as a background in cooking, I had never cooked anything before I started keto, but I had always loved *The Food Network* and cooking shows. I would study cooking techniques by watching and learning from them. I then adapted the recipes I saw them creating, into carnivore forms. Through trial and error, I perfected them.

Today, my son actually prefers my carnivore versions of his favorites as opposed to the fast-food and pre-packaged ones. It is my hope that you and your family will fall in love with them as well when you taste how incredibly delicious they are. They're nourishing, healthy, and work for your body instead of against it!

The Ultimate Carnivore Cookbook
www.bioptimizedketo.com

TABLE OF CONTENTS

Buffalo Chicken Sandwich 3
Rotisserie Grilled Pork Loin 4
Air Fried Beef Short Rib 6
Smoked Brisket 7
Grilled Flanken Cut Short Ribs 8
Chicken Fried Bacon 9
Chicken Pizza Pocket 11
Chicken Cutlet 13
Air Fried Lamb T-Bones 15
Air Fried Pork Belly 16
Simple Stuffed Bacon Cheeseburger 18
Chicken Heart Frittata (Dairy-Free) 20
Beef Liver Meatballs 22
Bacon Wrapped Meatloaf 24
Air Fried Lamb Meatballs 26
Boneless Fried Chicken Bites 28
Fried Mozzarella Sticks 30
Breakfast Sausage 32
Sweetbreads With White Gravy 33
Halloumi Fries 35
Chili Dogs on Carnivore Buns 36
Pressure Cooker Pulled Pork 39
Tacos de Lengua (Beef Tongue Tacos) 41
Organ Power Soup 43
Pan Seared Duck Breast 45
Paffle Pizza 47
Pâté "Corn" Puffs 48
Grilled Lamb Sweetbreads 51
Smoked Pork Tenderloin 53
Air Fried Cod Fillet 54
"Corn" Dogs 55
Garlic Butter Prime Rib 57
Air Fried Shrimp 59
Roasted Chicken 60
Bacon Wrapped Chicken Skewers 62
Smoked Pork Belly 64

TABLE OF CONTENTS

Garlic Parmesan Drumsticks 65
Mollejas Taco 67
Dairy-Free Chicken Pizza Crust 69
Parmesan Pork 71
Air Fried Chicken Tenders 73
Bacon Fat Chicken Liver Pâté 74
Steak Tacos 75
Oven Roasted Baby Back Ribs 77
Chicken & Cheese Pizza Crust 79
Roasted Bone Marrow 81
Smoked Veal Shanks 82
Pan Seared Egg Yolks 83
Herb Crusted Lamb Chops 85
Crunchy Cheese Shell Tacos 87
Beef Wellington 89
Bacon Wrapped Strip Steak 91
Primal Blend Burger..93
Sliced Beef Tongue 95
Bacon Wrapped Kidney Meatballs 97
Salmon Dip 99
Carnivore Bread 100
Carnivore Tortillas 102
Carnivore Noodles (Dairy-Free) 104
Carnivore Burger Bun 106
3 Cheese Butter 108
Carnivore Mayonnaise 110
Spicy Mayonnaise 111
Garlic Ghee 112
Garlic Hollandaise Sauce...113
Ranch Dressing 114
Beef Bone Broth 115
Carnivore-ish Chocolate Chip Waffles 116
Carnivore-ish French Toast Sticks 117
Carnivore Taffy 119
Carnivore-ish Cinnamon Roll 121
Carnivore-ish Brownie 123

BUFFALO CHICKEN SANDWICH

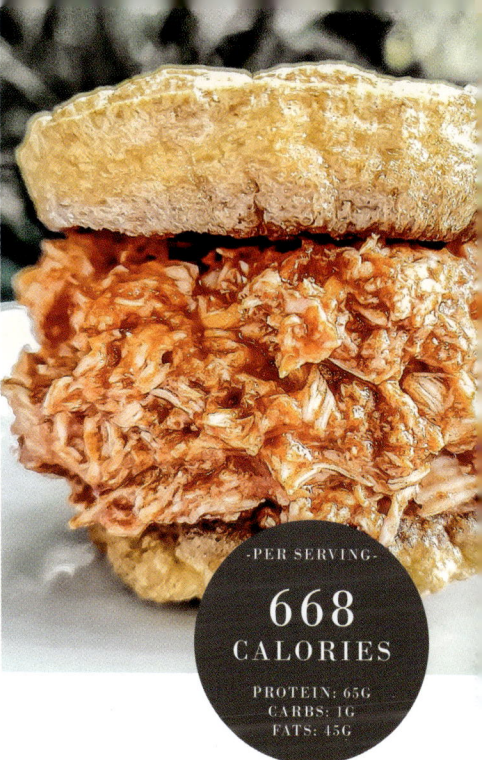

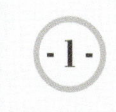  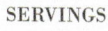

DIFFICULTY: -1-
SERVINGS: 4
TIME: PREPARATION 20 MINS / COOKING 25 MINS

-PER SERVING-
668 CALORIES
PROTEIN: 65G
CARBS: 1G
FATS: 45G

INGREDIENTS

1lb of Chicken Breasts
1 Tsp of Redmond Real Salt
1 Tbsp of Fat of Choice

1½ Cups of Carnivore Mayo* (see recipe)
1-2 Tbsp of Hot Sauce of Choice
Carnivore Bun* (see recipe)

STEPS

- 1 - Start by cooking the chicken breasts in a nonstick pan with 1 tbsp of fat searing the breasts until fully cooked.

- 2 - Remove from the pan and set aside to cool.

- 3 - Once cooled shred the breast meat and add to a large bowl.

- 4 - Put the carnivore mayo* into a separate bowl. Add the hot sauce into the mayo and mix together.

- 5 - Add the sauce to the shredded breast meat and stir thoroughly.

- 6 - Place on top of a Carnivore Bun.* (See recipe)

The Ultimate Carnivore Cookbook / 3
www.bioptimizedketo.com

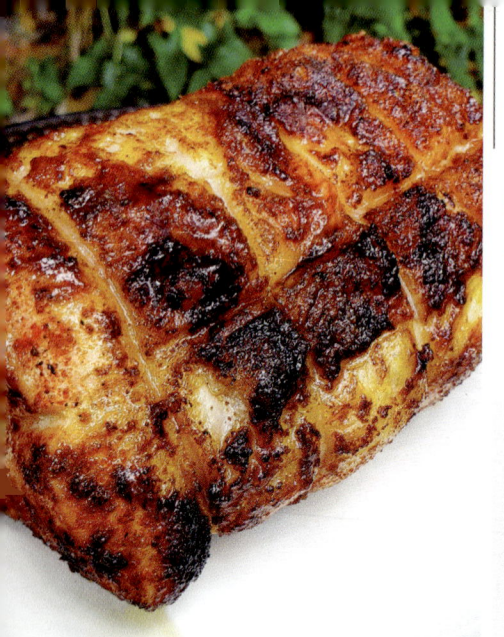

ROTISSERIE GRILLED PORK LOIN

TIME — PREPARATION 20 MINS, COOKING 2 HOURS

SERVINGS — 4

DIFFICULTY — 2

-PER SERVING-
518 CALORIES
PROTEIN: 75G
CARBS: 1G
FATS: 24G

INGREDIENTS

3 Lbs of Boneless Pork Loin Roast
2 Tsp of Redmond Real Salt
2 Tsp of Fresh Cracked Black Pepper
1½ Tsp of Paprika

STEPS

- 1 - Start by heating your grill to 350°F.

- 2 - While the grill is heating, skewer the pork loin onto the spit. Season with the salt, pepper, and paprika after it has been skewered.

- 3 - This will help prevent rubbing any seasonings off if you try to skewer after seasoning.

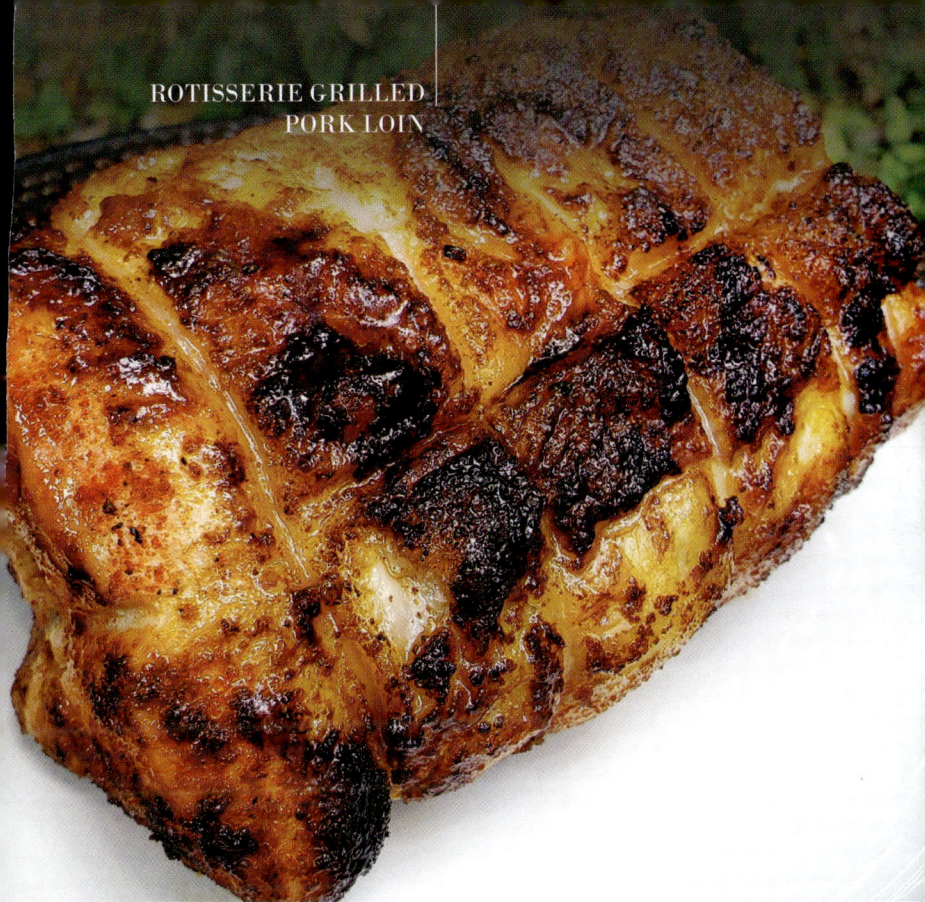

ROTISSERIE GRILLED PORK LOIN

STEPS

- 4 - To season, sprinkle the salt onto the entire loin, top, bottom, and sides. Then repeat with the black pepper. Lastly, coat and lightly rub with the paprika making the pork loin red on all sides.

- 5 - Place spit onto the rotisserie and leave rotating for 2 hours or when the internal temp has reached 175°F.

- 6 - When finished the loin should be lightly crispy on the fat side and juicy in the meat.

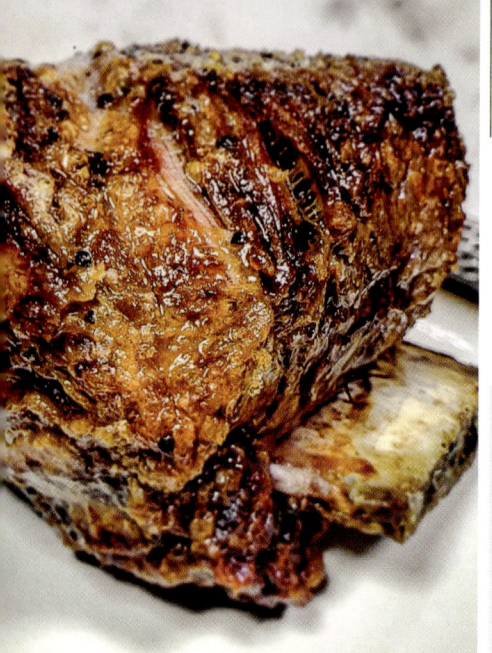

AIR FRIED BEEF SHORT RIB

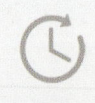

TIME
PREPARATION
10 MINS
COOKING
1 HOUR

SERVINGS
3

DIFFICULTY

-PER SERVING-
508 CALORIES
PROTEIN: 30G
CARBS: 0G
FATS: 29G

INGREDIENTS

1½ Lbs of Short Ribs
1½ Tsp of Redmond Real Salt
1 Tsp of Fresh Cracked Black Pepper

STEPS

- 1 - Season short ribs with salt and pepper being sure to coat all sides thoroughly.

- 2 - Heat your air fryer to 390°F.

- 3 - Once the air fryer reaches that temperature, place short ribs in about an inch apart.

- 4 - Cook for 45 minutes.

- 5 - Let rest for 15 minutes after cooking and then serve.

SMOKED BRISKET

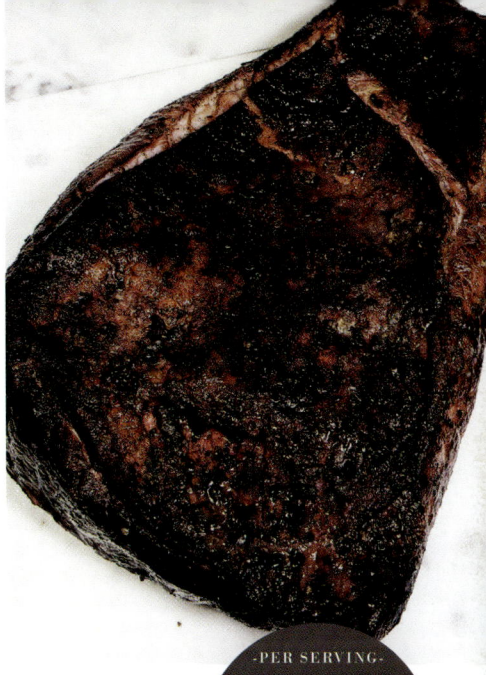

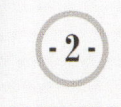
DIFFICULTY

SERVINGS
6

TIME
PREPARATION
15 MINS

COOKING
2-3 HOURS

-PER SERVING-
537 CALORIES
PROTEIN: 97G
CARBS: 0G
FATS: 16G

INGREDIENTS

6 Lbs Flat Cut Brisket
1-2 Tsp of Redmond Real Salt
1½ Tsp of Fresh Cracked Black Pepper

STEPS

- 1 - Season the whole brisket with the salt and pepper starting with the bottom and then flipping to season the top.

- 2 - Start a strong fire in the smoker until it's 250°F.

- 3 - Place the brisket on the far side from the fire.

- 4 - Cook until the internal temperature of the brisket reaches 200°F and pull from the smoker.

- 5 - Wrap the brisket in butchers paper and let rest for at least an hour before slicing.

The Ultimate Carnivore Cookbook / 7
www.bioptimizedketo.com

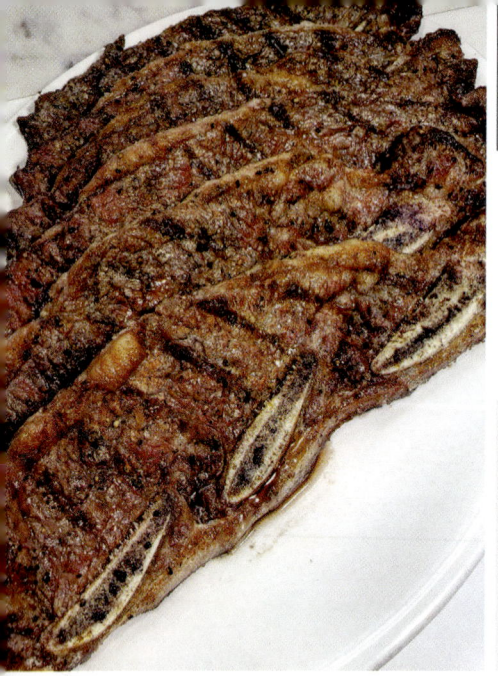

GRILLED FLANKEN CUT SHORT RIBS

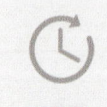 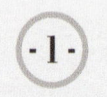

TIME — PREPARATION 15 MINS / COOKING 10 MINS
SERVINGS — 4
DIFFICULTY — 1

-PER SERVING-
508 CALORIES
PROTEIN: 41G
CARBS: 0G
FATS: 38G

INGREDIENTS

1½ Lbs of Flanken Cut Short Ribs
1½ Tsp of Redmond Real Salt
1 Tsp of Fresh Cracked Black Pepper

STEPS

- 1 - Preheat the grill to 350°F.

- 2 - Season both sides of the ribs with salt and pepper.

- 3 - Place on the grill and cook for 5 minutes on each side with the grill open.

    Note Thinner cuts may cook quicker or lose the end bone.

CHICKEN FRIED BACON

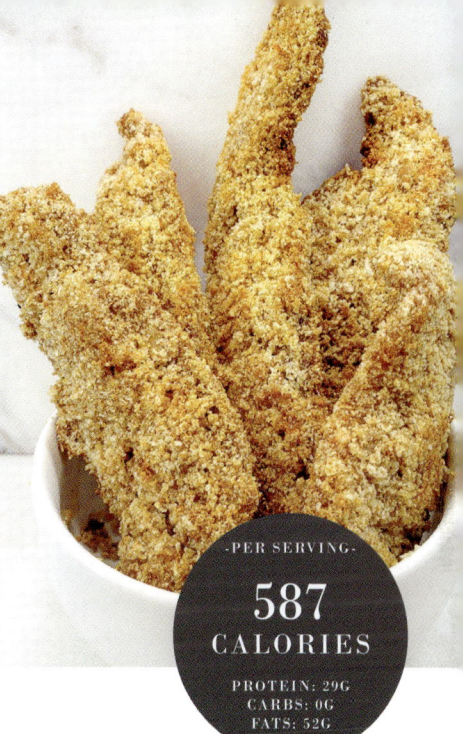

DIFFICULTY
- 2 -

SERVINGS
4

TIME
PREPARATION
35 MINS
COOKING
30 MINS

-PER SERVING-
587 CALORIES
PROTEIN: 29G
CARBS: 0G
FATS: 52G

INGREDIENTS

1 8 Oz Pack of Sugar-Free Bacon
1 Cup of Pork Panko by Bacon's Heir
1 Tsp of Redmond Real Salt

2 Cups of Fat of Choice
2 Large Eggs

STEPS

- 1 - Lightly pre-cook the bacon any way that is comfortable (e.g. fried or baked).

    Note The bacon should still be bendy and not crunchy.

- 2 - Crack and scramble the 2 large eggs in a wide bowl.

    Note If a wide bowl is unavailable, cut bacon strips in half for easier coating.

- 3 - Mix Pork Panko and salt together in a separate bowl.

- 4 - One piece at a time, soak bacon in the eggs then roll in the Pork Panko.

The Ultimate Carnivore Cookbook / 9
www.bioptimizedketo.com

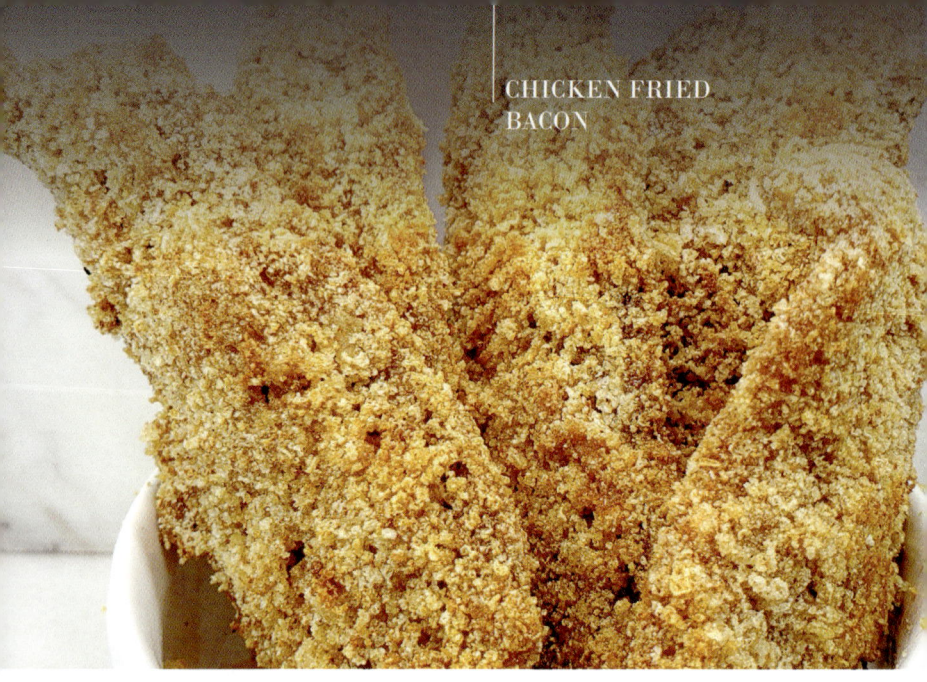

CHICKEN FRIED BACON

STEPS

- 5 - Move from the Pork Panko bowl and back into the egg bowl being careful to not wash off the coating.

- 6 - Place back into the Pork Panko bowl for a second coat and then set to the side until these steps have been completed for all pieces of bacon.

- 7 - Heat a pot with your fat of choice to medium-high heat.

- 8 - Once the pot of fat has heated, place the now coated bacon into the pot to fry.

- 9 - Cook until the coating becomes a golden brown and is crispy.

    Note Do not try to fry too many pieces at once. Depending upon the size of the pot, it may be necessary to do them in batches of 3 to 5 pieces at a time.

- 10 - Remove from the pot and place on a cooling rack for a few minutes while you finish cooking the rest.

CHICKEN PIZZA POCKET

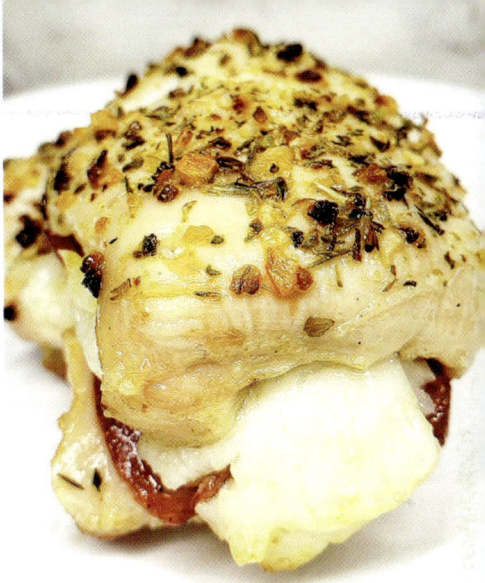

DIFFICULTY

SERVINGS
2

TIME
PREPARATION
25 MINS
COOKING
30 MINS

-PER SERVING-
303 CALORIES
PROTEIN: 34G
CARBS: 0G
FATS: 19G

INGREDIENTS

1 Chicken Breast
3 1 Oz Balls of Fresh Mozzarella
5-10 Pepperoni Slices
½ Tsp of Redmond Real Salt
1 Tsp of Garlic & Herb Seasoning
¼ Tsp of Pizza Season (Optional)

STEPS

- 1 -   Preheat the oven to 350°F.

- 2 -   Pat dry the chicken breast and carefully cut a pocket into it as deep as you can without cutting through the side, bottom, or back.

- 3 -   Line the pepperoni on the inside of the breast and then stuff with the mozzarella balls.

The Ultimate Carnivore Cookbook / 11
www.bioptimizedketo.com

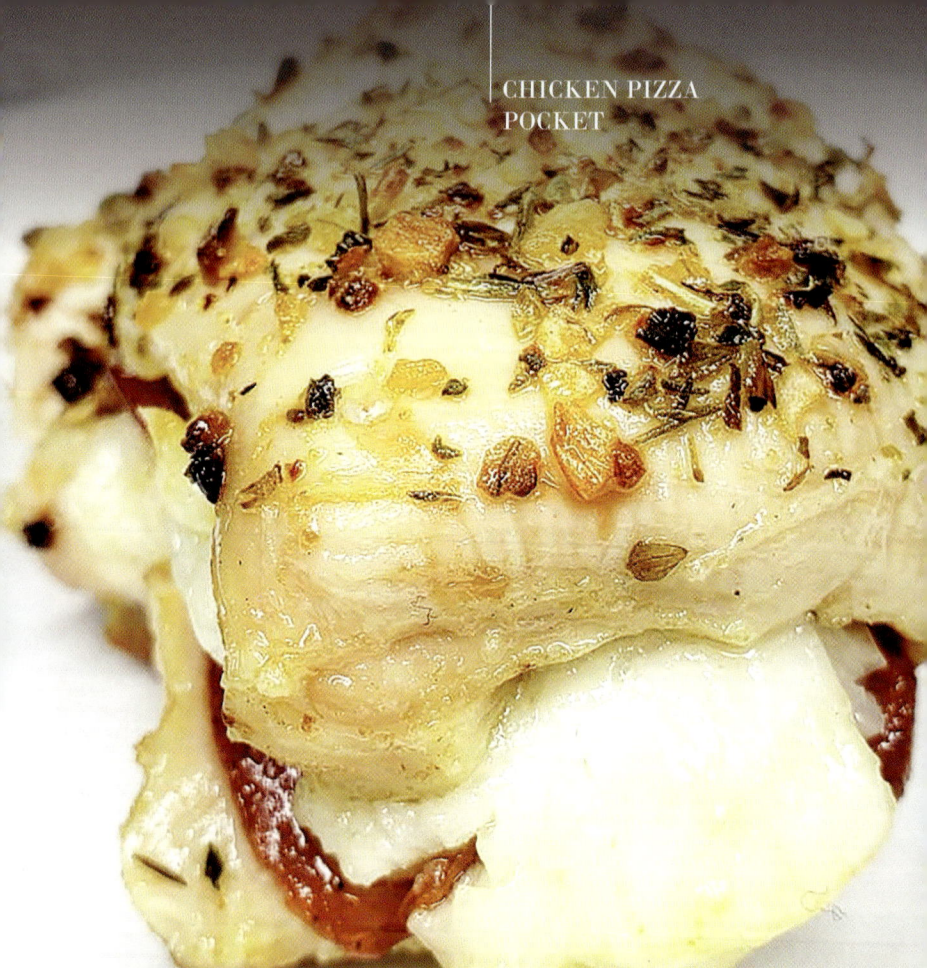

CHICKEN PIZZA POCKET

STEPS

Note It helps to fit the pepperoni and cheese easier inside by squeezing the chicken breast slightly to round and open the hole.

- 4 - Season the outside with garlic & herb seasoning and pizza seasoning.

- 5 - Place onto a baking sheet lined with parchment paper and bake in the oven for 25-30 minutes or until internal temperature reaches a minimum of 165°F.

CHICKEN CUTLET

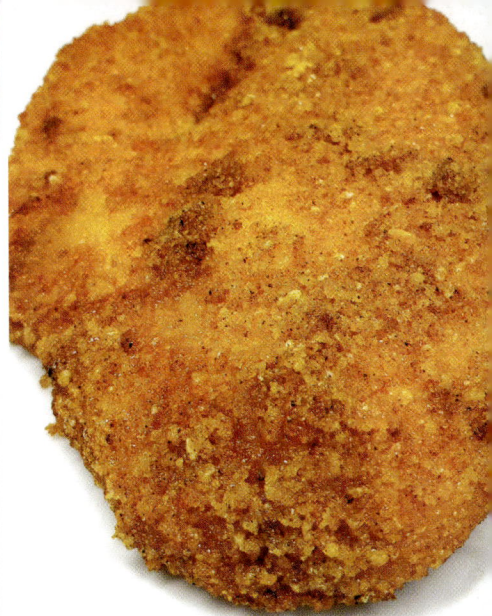

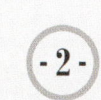 

DIFFICULTY: 2
SERVINGS: 1
TIME: PREPARATION 20 MINS / COOKING 25 MINS

-PER SERVING-
1629 CALORIES
PROTEIN: 145G
CARBS: 2G
FATS: 116G

INGREDIENTS

1 Chicken Breast (approximately ½ Lb)
1 Tsp of Paprika
1 Tsp of Redmond Real Salt
1 Tsp of Fresh Cracked Black Pepper
1 Cup of Pork Panko by Bacon's Heir
2 Large Eggs
2 Tbsp of Fat of Choice

STEPS

- 1 - Start by taking the chicken breast and using a meat tenderizer, pound it flat until it is about 1/4 of an inch thick.

- 2 - Season both sides with salt and pepper.

- 3 - Next put the Pork Panko in a bowl and add salt, pepper, and paprika to it and mix together.

- 4 - Crack and scramble the 2 large eggs into a separate bowl.

The Ultimate Carnivore Cookbook / 13
www.bioptimizedketo.com

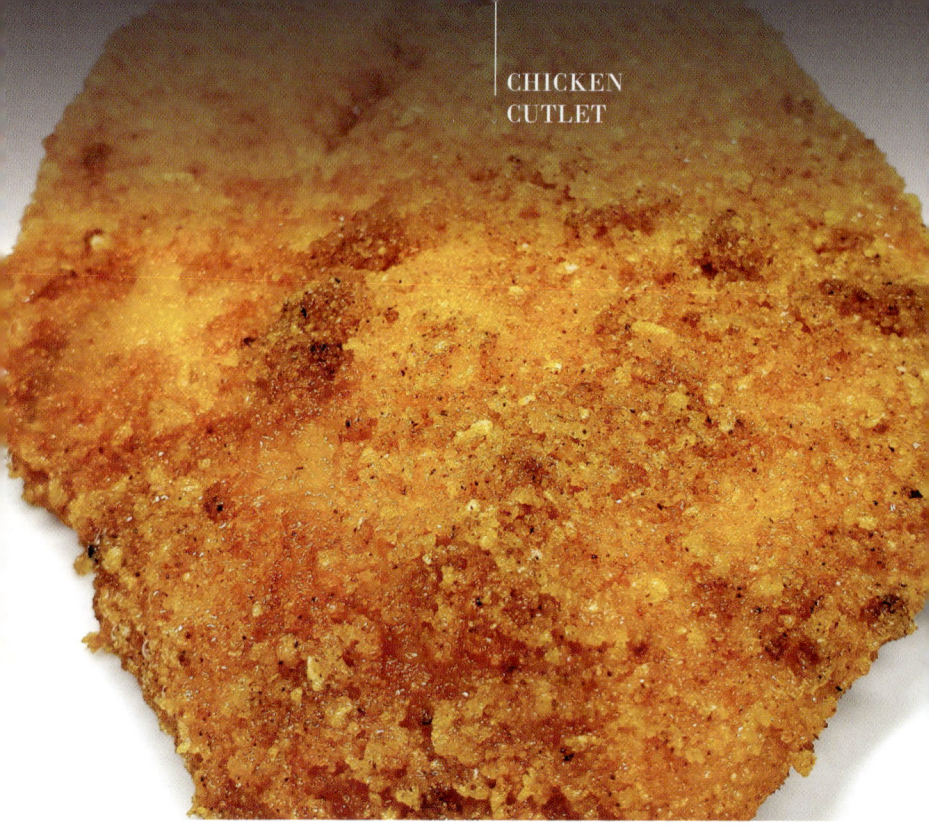

CHICKEN CUTLET

STEPS

- 5 - Dip the flattened chicken breast into the beaten eggs and then move into the Pork Panko coating both sides.

- 6 - Place cutlet to the side until ready to cook.

- 7 - Preheat the oven to 400°F.

- 8 - Place your fat of choice onto a baking sheet lined with aluminum foil and put it into the oven for 5 minutes to melt the fat.

- 9 - Once the fat has melted, place the cutlet onto the baking sheet and put it into the oven for 20 minutes.

- 10 - After the 20 minutes, remove from the oven and rest on a cooling rack.

AIR FRIED LAMB T-BONES

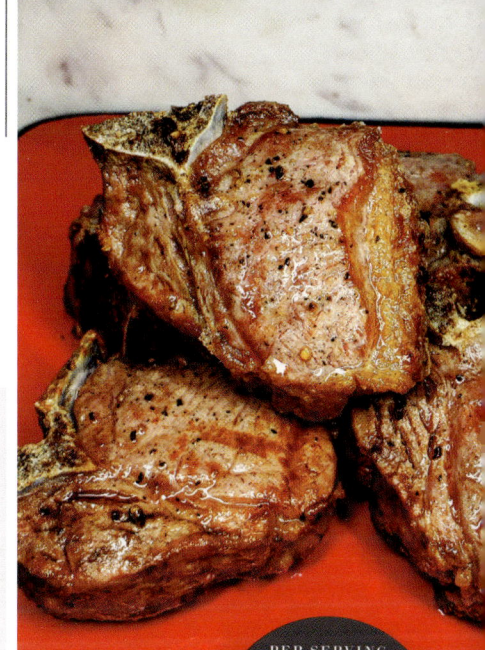

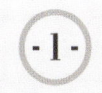
DIFFICULTY

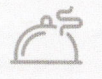
SERVINGS
2

TIME
PREPARATION
15 MINS
COOKING
10 MINS

-PER SERVING-
473 CALORIES
PROTEIN: 29G
CARBS: 0G
FATS: 40G

INGREDIENTS

5 Lamb T-Bones also called Loin Chops (approximately 72 grams each)
1½ Tsp of Redmond Real Salt
1 Tsp of Fresh Cracked Black Pepper

STEPS

- 1 - Lay out the lamb T-Bones on a preparation board or piece of parchment paper to be seasoned.

- 2 - Sprinkle salt and pepper on both sides of the T-Bones and then roll the fat caps of each one in the excess salt and pepper that is left on the board or parchment paper.

- 3 - Preheat the air fryer to 390°F.

- 4 - After the air fryer has reached the temperature, place the T-Bones in and cook for 10 minutes flipping them halfway through the cook.

The Ultimate Carnivore Cookbook / 15
www.bioptimizedketo.com

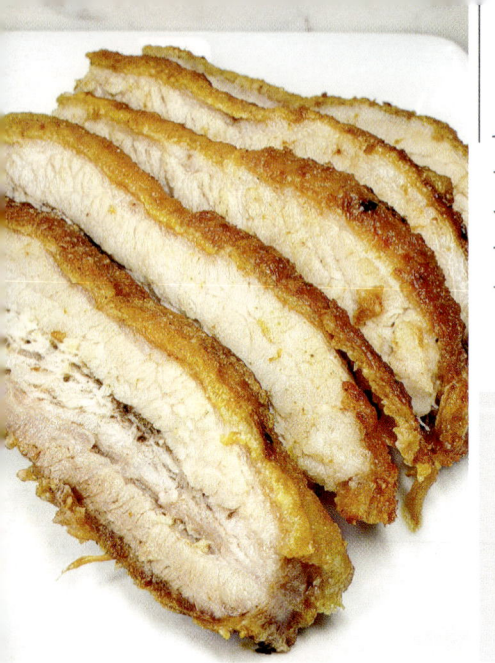

AIR FRIED PORK BELLY

TIME
PREPARATION
3-6 HOURS
COOKING
55 MINS

SERVINGS
6

DIFFICULTY

-PER SERVING-
1167 CALORIES
PROTEIN: 21G
CARBS: 0G
FATS: 120G

INGREDIENTS

3 Lbs Slab of Pork Belly
1 Tbsp of Redmond Real Salt

STEPS

- 1 - Start by pat drying the pork belly and then layering salt evenly on top of the skin.

- 2 - Let sit on a wire rack in the refrigerator for 3 to 6 hours.

- 3 - The salt will pull any excess moisture from the skin.

- 4 - Once ready for cooking remove the salt layer and score lengthwise about a half inch apart.

- 5 - Preheat the air fryer to 450°F.

- 6 - Sprinkle the skin with a thin layer of salt this time.

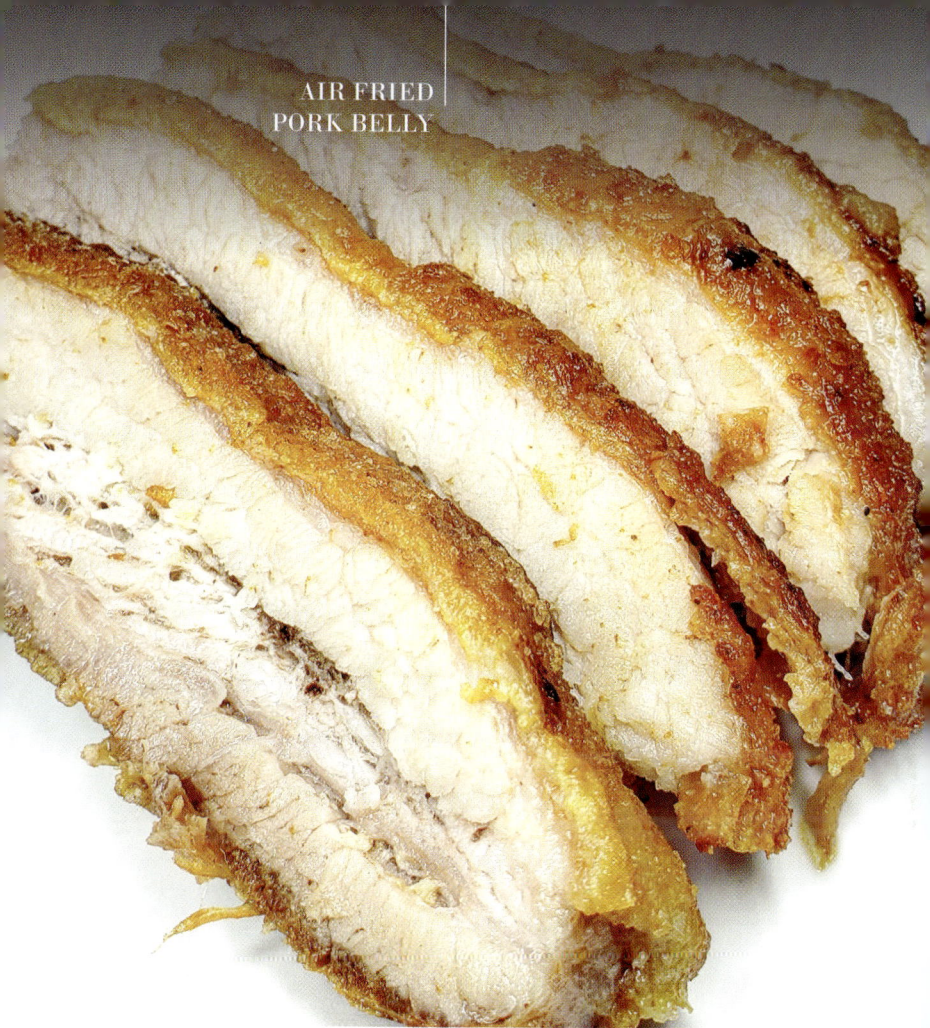

AIR FRIED PORK BELLY

STEPS

- 7 - Place pork belly into the air fryer.

- 8 - Cook at this temp for 35 minutes or until the skin has browned and started to develop crispy bumps.

- 9 - Turn heat down to 325°F and cook for an additional 25 minutes.

- 10 - Remove from the air fryer and slice along the score marks.

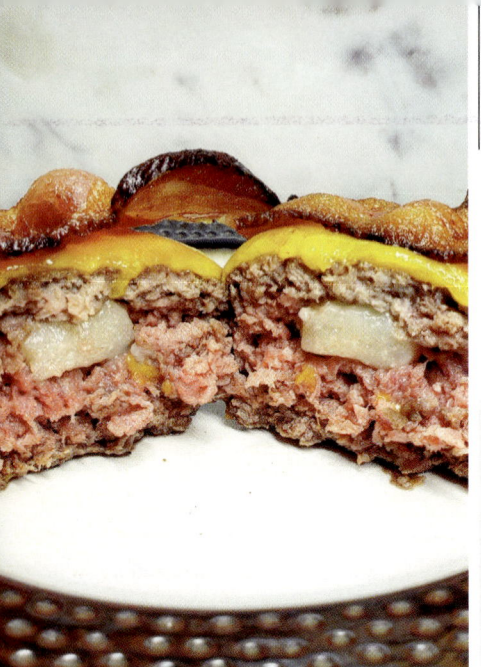

SIMPLE STUFFED BACON CHEESEBURGER

TIME	SERVINGS	DIFFICULTY
PREPARATION 20 MINS	4	-1-
COOKING 10-20 MINS		

-PER SERVING-

601 CALORIES

PROTEIN: 36G
CARBS: 2G
FATS: 50G

INGREDIENTS

- 1 Lb of Ground Beef (85/15)
- 4 Oz of a Hard Cheese
- 2 Slices of Cheddar Cheese
- 1 Tsp of Redmond Real Salt
- ½ Tsp of Fresh Cracked Black Pepper
- 1 8 Oz Pack of Sugar-Free Bacon

STEPS

- 1 - Place ground beef on a sheet of parchment paper and press it into a flat square.

- 2 - Season with salt and pepper and then cut the square in half.

- 3 - Roll each half into a ball.

- 4 - Cut the hard cheese into ½ inch thick squares and place one inside of each burger ball.

SIMPLE STUFFED BACON CHEESEBURGER

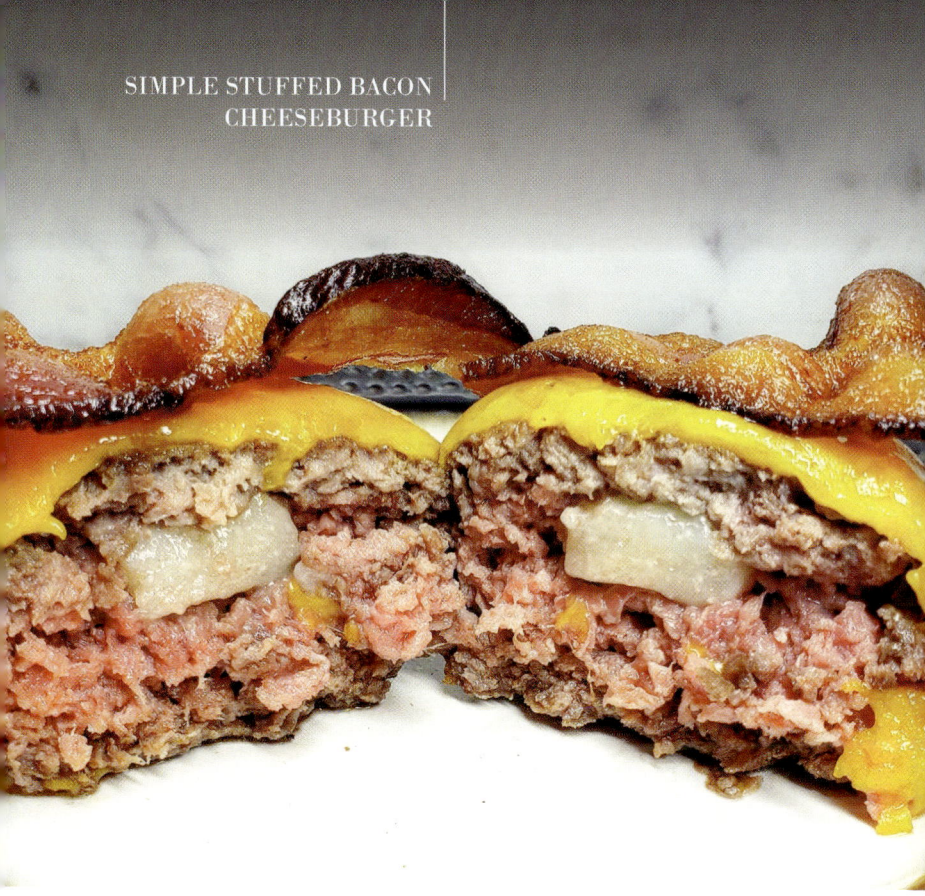

STEPS

- 5 - Preheat the grill to 350°F.

- 6 - Press the balls down lightly creating a flat top and bottom.

- 7 - Place the burgers on to the grill and cook each side with the top open for 5 minutes for a medium rare burger or 10 minutes for a well done burger.

- 8 - Once cooked, turn the burners off and place slices of cheese on top of the burgers and close the top allowing the cheese to melt inside of the grill.

- 9 - Top with bacon.

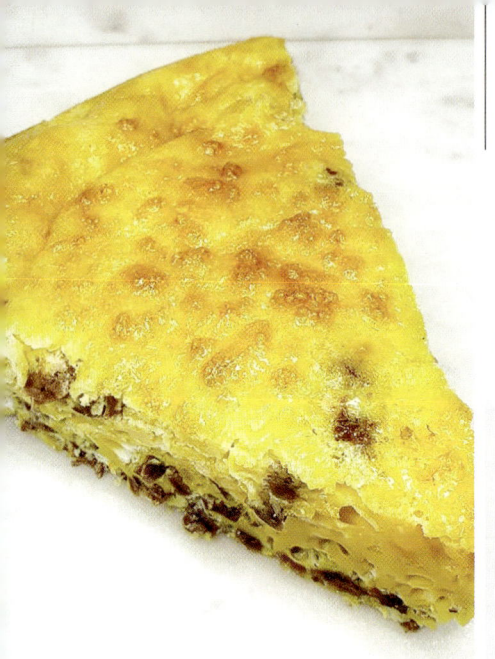

CHICKEN HEART FRITTATA
(DAIRY-FREE)

TIME   **SERVINGS**   **DIFFICULTY**

PREPARATION   6
20 MINS

COOKING
45 MINS

-PER SERVING-

471 CALORIES

PROTEIN: 49G
CARBS: 2G
FATS: 30G

INGREDIENTS

3 Tablespoons of Fat of Choice
1½ Lbs of Chicken Hearts
2 Tsp of Redmond Real Salt
18 Large Eggs

STEPS

- 1 -   Begin by heating a cast iron skillet or a deep nonstick pan to medium-high heat with the fat.

- 2 -   Once heated, add in the chicken hearts and fry until browned on both sides.

- 3 -   Leaving the fat in the pan, remove the hearts from the pan and set to the side to cool.

- 4 -   Preheat the oven to 350°F.

CHICKEN HEART FRITTATA
(DAIRY-FREE)

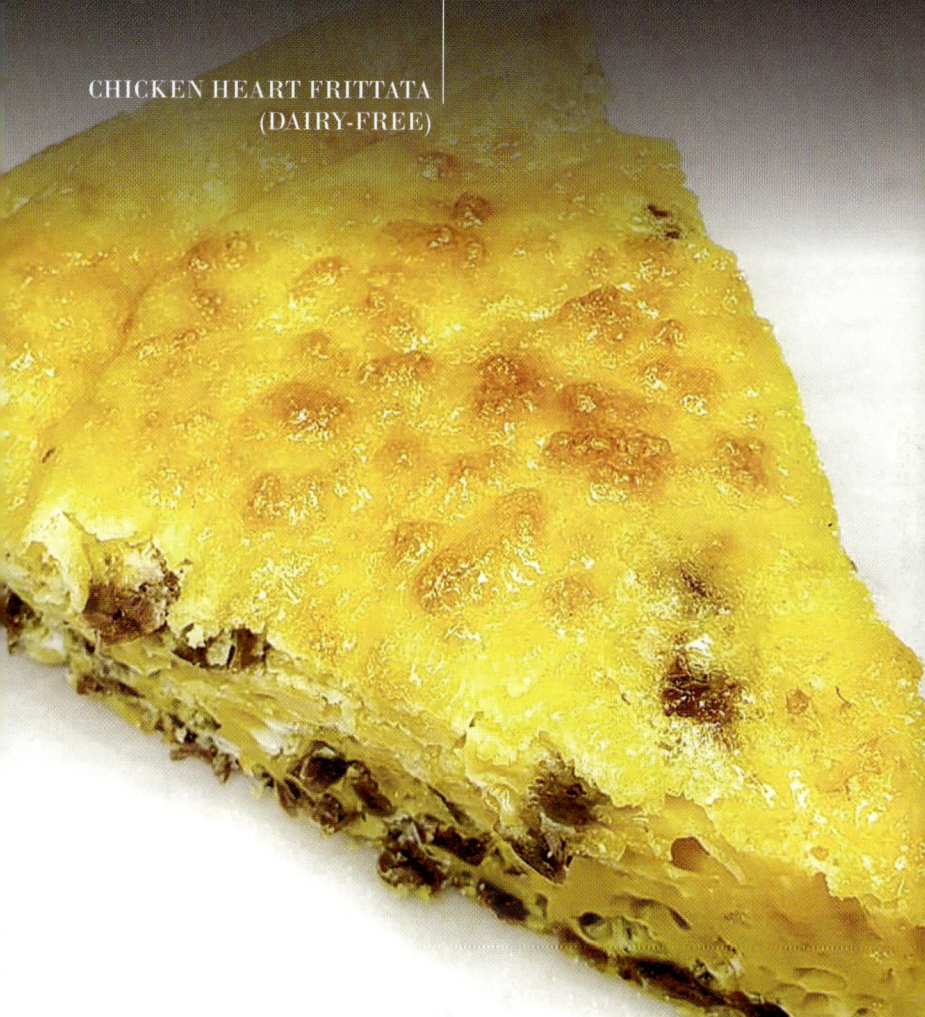

STEPS

- 5 -   Once the pan has cooled, begin cracking the 18 eggs into the pan and then scramble them with the fat that is still in the pan.

- 6 -   Chop the hearts into small pieces and add to the eggs.

- 7 -   Add salt and stir together.

- 8 -   Place into the oven and bake for 25 minutes.

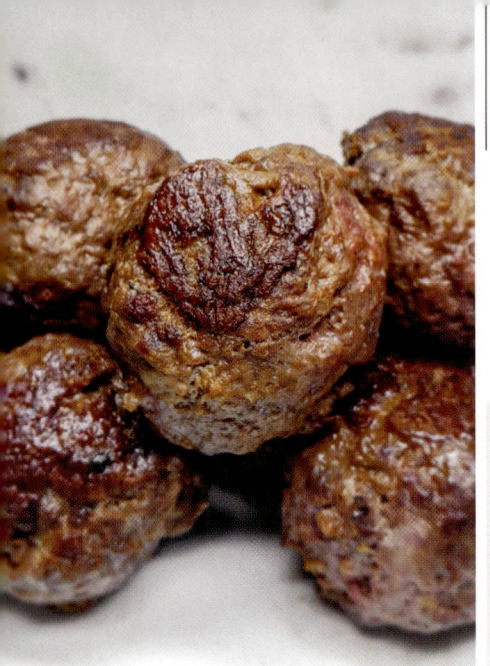

BEEF LIVER MEATBALLS

TIME   **SERVINGS**   **DIFFICULTY**

PREPARATION   6
35 MINS

COOKING
25 MINS

-PER SERVING-
493 CALORIES

PROTEIN: 50G
CARBS: 3G
FATS: 31G

INGREDIENTS

- 2 Lbs of Ground Beef (85/15)
- 1 Lb of Beef Liver
- 3 Tsp of Redmond Real Salt
- 1½ Tsp of Fresh Cracked Black Pepper
- 2 Tsp of Ground Cumin (Optional)
- 2 Tbsp of Fat of Choice

STEPS

- 1 - Slice liver into strips.

- 2 - Place liver in a food processor and lightly grind down.

- 3 - Add the liver into 2 pounds of ground beef in a large bowl and mix thoroughly.

- 4 - Press the meat blend between 2 pieces of parchment and roll flat to about an inch thick.

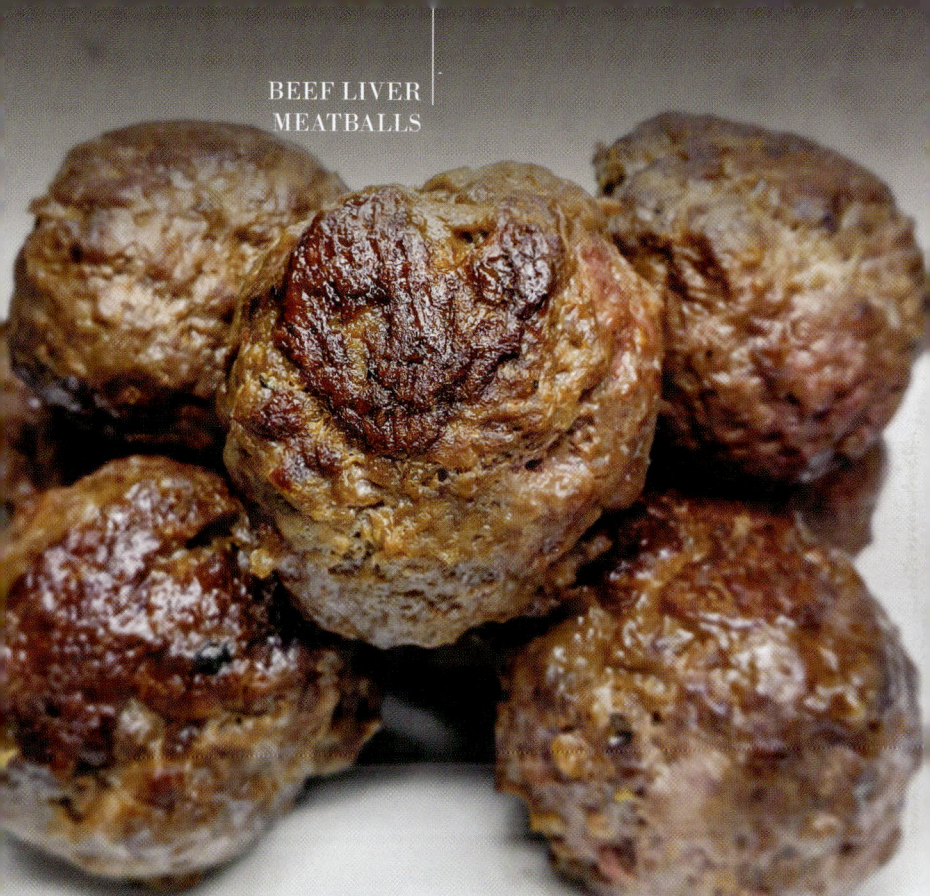

BEEF LIVER MEATBALLS

STEPS

- 5 - Season with salt, pepper and ground cumin.

    Note Ground cumin can be great for masking the bold liver but its not necessary.

- 6 - After seasoning, pinch a few ounces off and roll into balls.

- 7 - Heat a cast-iron skillet or nonstick pan to medium-high heat.

- 8 - Add fat of choice and place meatballs into the pan.

- 9 - Cook and turn until the sides have browned and created a light crust.

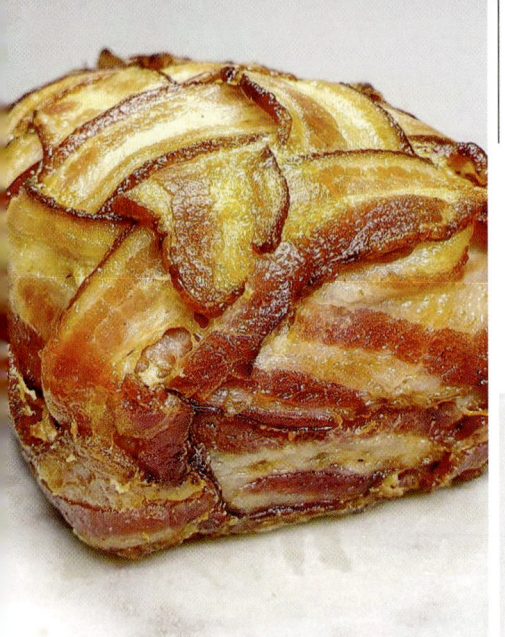

BACON WRAPPED MEATLOAF

 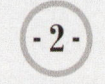

TIME
PREPARATION
25 MINS
COOKING
1¼ HOURS

SERVINGS
8

DIFFICULTY

-PER SERVING-
591 CALORIES
PROTEIN: 43G
CARBS: 0G
FATS: 46G

INGREDIENTS

2 8 Oz Packs of Sugar-Free Bacon
2 Lbs of Ground Beef (85/15)
8 Ounces of Sugar Free Diced Ham
8 Tbsp of Pork Panko by Bacon's Heir
2 Large Eggs
1½ Tsp of Redmond Real Salt
1 Tsp of Fresh Cracked Pepper

STEPS

- 1 - Preheat oven to 400°F.

- 2 - Add all ingredients (except for bacon) together in large mixing bowl and mix thoroughly.

- 3 - Lay bacon on a piece of parchment and create a weave.

BACON WRAPPED MEATLOAF

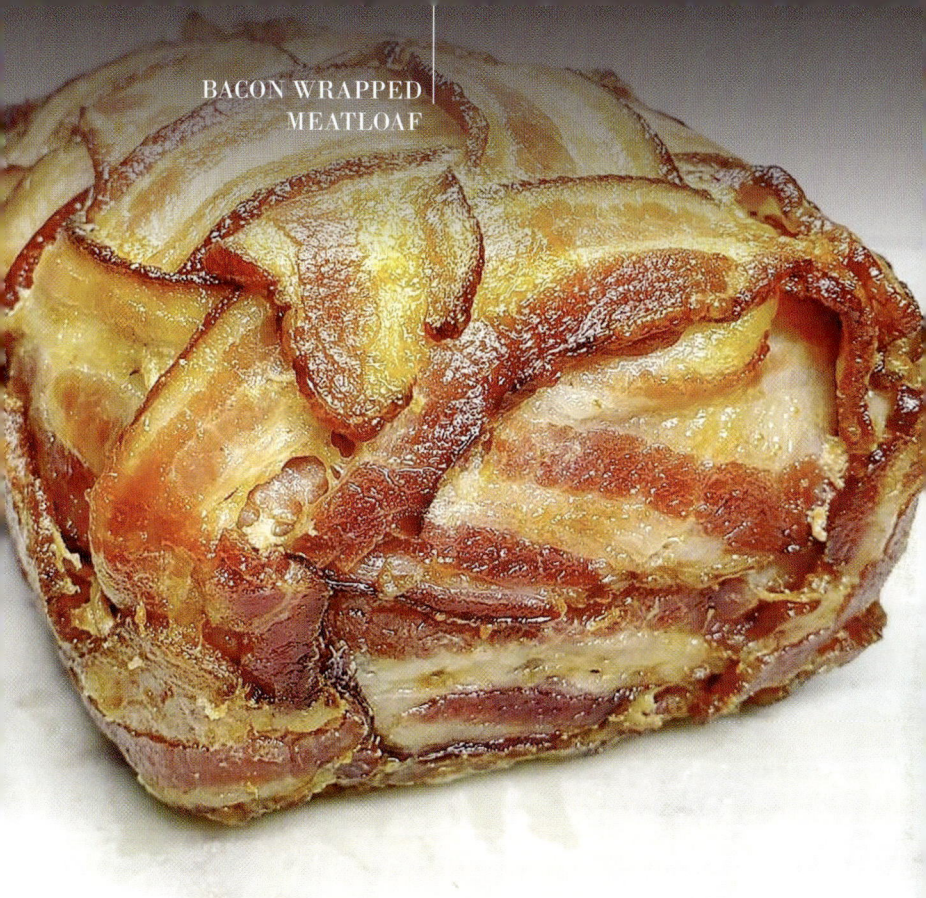

STEPS

- 4 - Pack meatloaf mix tightly together and place in the center of the weaved bacon.

- 5 - Wrap the bacon tightly over the meat mixture and close the ends.

- 6 - Place the wrapped meatloaf into a standard loaf pan.

- 7 - Place into the oven and cook for 75 minutes.

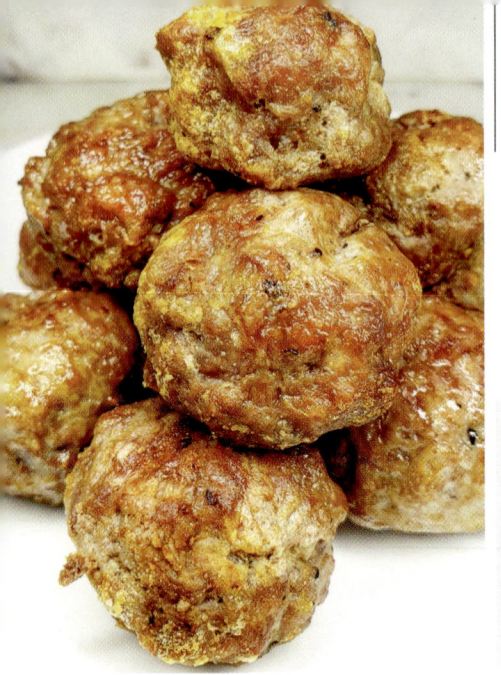

AIR FRIED LAMB MEATBALLS

 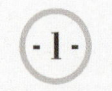

TIME   **SERVINGS**   **DIFFICULTY**

PREPARATION
20 MINS

COOKING
10 MINS

2

-PER SERVING-

714 CALORIES

PROTEIN: 42G
CARBS: 0G
FATS: 61G

INGREDIENTS

1 Lb of Ground Lamb
1½ Tbsp of Pork Panko by Bacon's Heir
1½ Tsp of Redmond Real Salt
½ Tsp of Fresh Cracked Black Pepper

STEPS

- 1 -   Unpack ground lamb into a bowl and mix in Pork Panko.

         Note If Pork Panko is not available this step can be skipped, meatballs may open up a bit during cooking though.

- 2 -   Press ground lamb thin on a piece of parchment.

- 3 -   Season with salt and pepper.

- 4 -   After seasoned, start pinching the lamb off into the desired size of meatball.

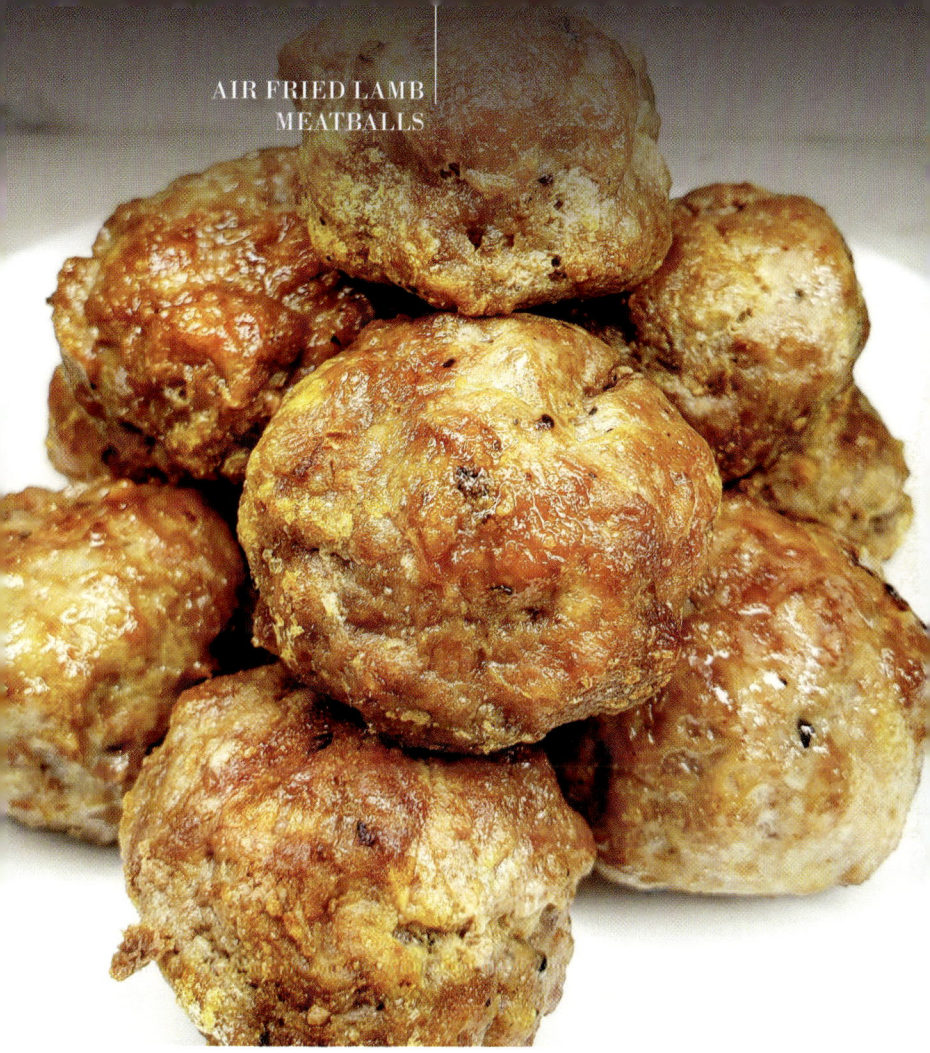

AIR FRIED LAMB MEATBALLS

STEPS

- 5 - Rolling in hands packing the meat firmly between your palms.
- 6 - Preheat the air fryer to 390°F.
- 7 - Cook for 10 minutes in the air fryer flipping at the halfway mark.
- 8 - Remove and serve.

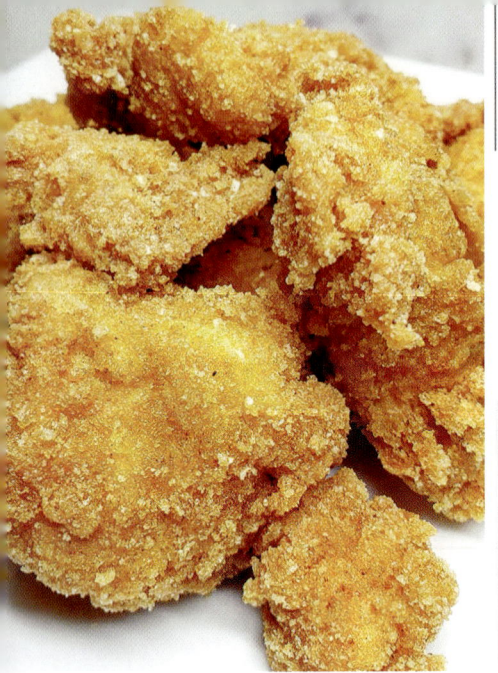

BONELESS FRIED CHICKEN BITES

TIME | **SERVINGS** | **DIFFICULTY**

PREPARATION
30 MINS

COOKING
40 MINS

3

-PER SERVING-

1087 CALORIES

PROTEIN: 112G
CARBS: 8G
FATS: 67G

INGREDIENTS

1 Lb of Chicken Breast
1 Cup of Whey Protein Isolate
1 Cup of Pork Panko by Bacon's Heir
2 Large Eggs
1 Tsp of Redmond Real Salt
4 Cups of Fat of Choice

STEPS

- 1 - Cut chicken breast into cubes.

- 2 - Salt the chicken and let sit for a few minutes.

- 3 - Bring a pot with fat of choice to medium-high heat on the stove.

- 4 - Using 3 separate bowls, crack the eggs in bowl number 1, the whey protein isolate in bowl number 2, and the Pork Panko into bowl number 3.

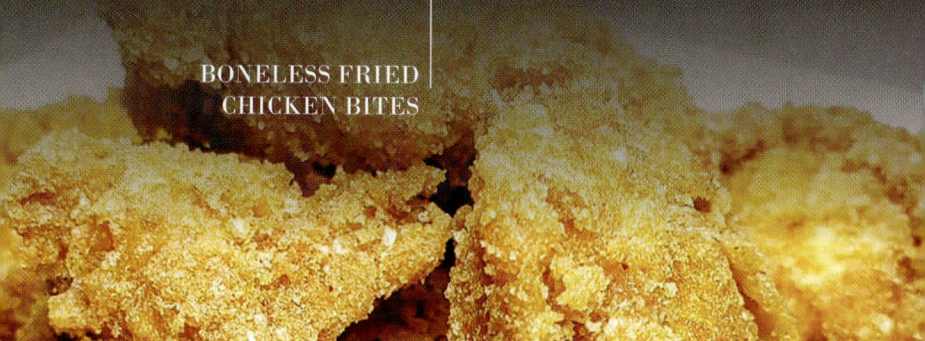

BONELESS FRIED CHICKEN BITES

STEPS

- 5 - Place chicken chunks into the eggs a few pieces at a time.

- 6 - Move from there to the bowl of whey protein isolate and roll until fully coated.

- 7 - Move the chunks back to the egg bowl and then into the Pork Panko rolling again until coated all around.

- 8 - Set aside until ready to fry.

- 9 - Repeat this for all the chicken chunks.

- 10 - Once all of the chicken chunks have gone through the double coating process, it's time to fry.

- 11 - The size of the pot chosen will determine how many pieces can be cooked at a time.

    Note Don't crowd the pot.

- 12 - I recommend there to be at least 1½ inch between each piece inside of the pot.

- 13 - While frying, move the chunks around the pot with a metal strainer and flip after 5 minutes of cooking.

- 14 - Cook for another 5 minutes or until the breading has developed a golden brown and crispy exterior.

- 15 - After cooking remove from the pot and set on a cooling rack.

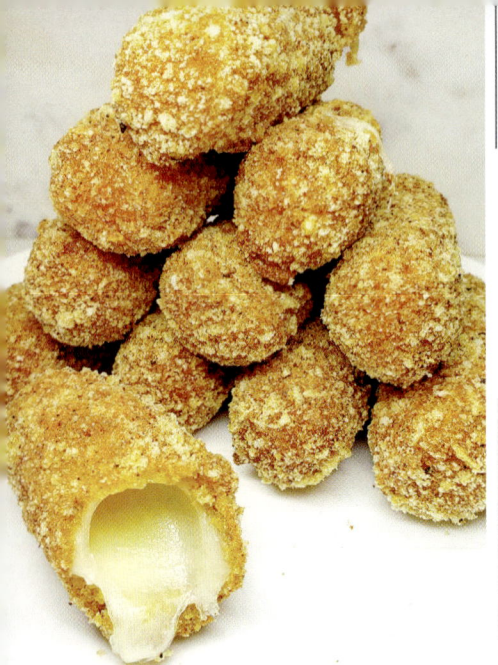

FRIED MOZZARELLA STICKS

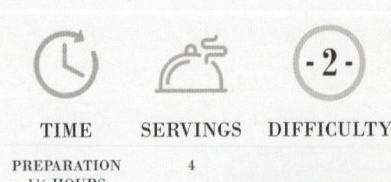

TIME
PREPARATION
1½ HOURS
COOKING
30 MINS

SERVINGS
4

DIFFICULTY
-2-

-PER SERVING-
832 CALORIES
PROTEIN: 59G
CARBS: 13G
FATS: 60G

INGREDIENTS

6 Mozzarella Sticks
2½ Cups of Pork Panko by Bacon's Heir
1½ Tbsp of Unflavored Whey Protein Isolate
1 Tsp of Paprika
1 Tsp of Redmond Real Salt
½ Tsp of Fresh Cracked Pepper
½ Tsp of Granulated Garlic
¼ Tsp of Granulated Onion
2 Large Eggs
2-3 Cups of Fat of Choice

STEPS

- 1 -   Start by mixing dry ingredients together in a bowl creating the breading mixture.

- 2 -   Crack and scramble the 2 eggs into a separate bowl.

- 3 -   Cut mozzarella sticks in half.

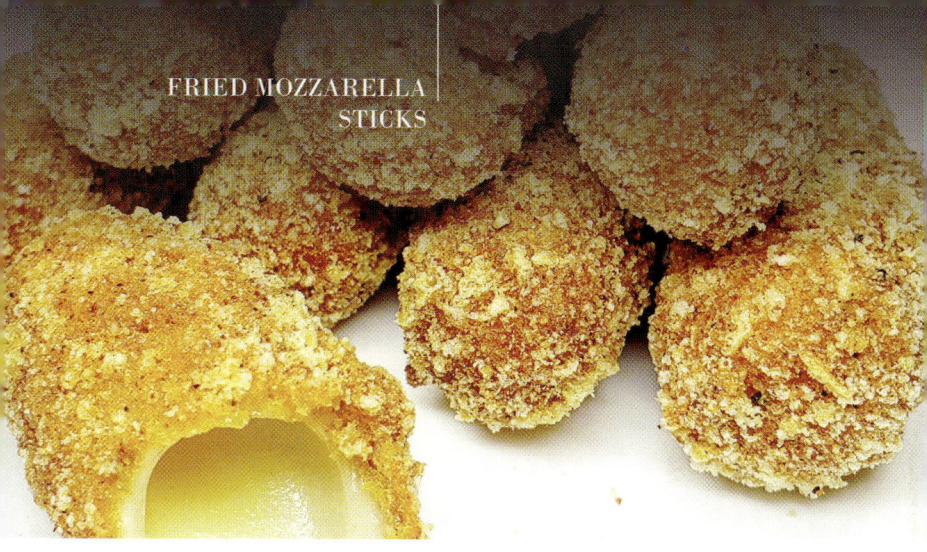

FRIED MOZZARELLA STICKS

STEPS

- 4 - One half stick at a time, dunk into the eggs and then roll in the breading bowl.

- 5 - After, gently return the breaded mozzarella stick to the egg bowl and carefully cover it with eggs.

    Note Be careful to not wash off the breading.

- 6 - Move mozzarella stick back to the breading for the final coating.

- 7 - Set to the side while completing this process to all mozzarella sticks.

- 8 - Freeze the mozzarella sticks for at least an hour before frying.

- 9 - When ready to fry, add fat to a pot and heat to medium-high heat.

    Note Fat should be at least 2 inches deep.

- 10 - Fry mozzarella sticks for 5 to 6 minutes or until golden brown and crispy.

- 11 - Set on a cooling rack for 3 minutes and serve immediately after.

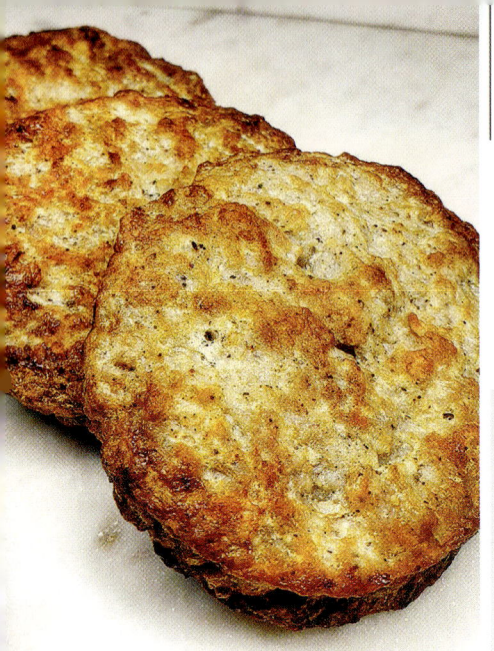

BREAKFAST SAUSAGE

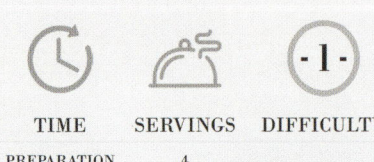

TIME
PREPARATION
20 MINS
COOKING
25 MINS

SERVINGS
4

DIFFICULTY
-1-

-PER SERVING-
327 CALORIES
PROTEIN: 20G
CARBS: 1G
FATS: 27G

INGREDIENTS

1 Lb of Ground Pork
1 Tsp of Redmond Real Salt
1 Tsp of Sage
1 Tsp Marjoram
¾ Tsp of Black Pepper
¼ Tsp of Allspice
¼ Tsp of Ground Nutmeg
1 Tbsp of Fat of Choice

STEPS

- 1 - Mix all ingredients together in a large bowl.

- 2 - Heat a cast iron skillet or nonstick pan to medium high heat with fat of choice.

- 3 - Form the sausage mixture into 1/4 inch thick patties.

  Note Can also be made into logs for sausage links.

- 4 - Cook patties in a pan with fat for 5 minutes or until the bottoms have caramelized.

- 5 - Flip patties over and cook for 5 more minutes.

SWEETBREADS WITH WHITE GRAVY

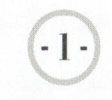  

DIFFICULTY - 1 -

SERVINGS 4

TIME
PREPARATION 40 MINS
COOKING 25 MINS

-PER SERVING-
488 CALORIES
PROTEIN: 30G
CARBS: 3G
FATS: 40G

INGREDIENTS

SWEETBREAD RECIPE

1 Lb of Veal Sweetbreads
1½ Tbsp of Butter or Ghee
1 Tsp of Redmond Real Salt

GRAVY RECIPE

1 Cup of Bone Broth* (see recipe)
1½ Cups of Heavy Cream
1 Tsp of Redmond Real Salt
1 Tsp of Fresh Cracked Black Pepper

STEPS

- 1 - Start blanching the sweetbreads by placing into a pot of cool water and bringing it to a boil.

- 2 - Once boiling, reduce heat to a simmer and continue blanching for 10 minutes.

- 3 - Remove the sweetbreads from the water and place into a bowl with ice and cold water for 30 minutes.

- 4 - Remove from the bowl and begin to pull or cut apart.

The Ultimate Carnivore Cookbook / 33
www.bioptimizedketo.com

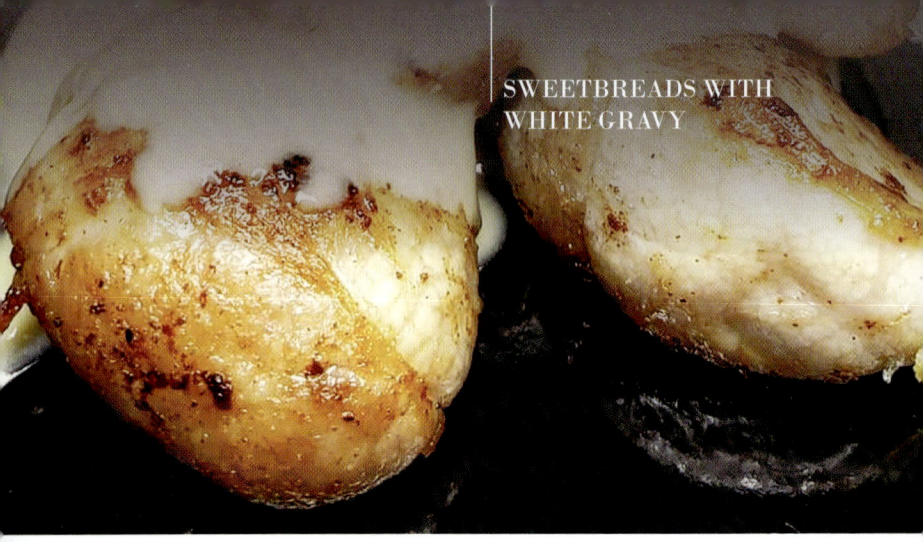

SWEETBREADS WITH WHITE GRAVY

STEPS

- 5 - Next, start making the gravy.

- 6 - Mix all gravy ingredients together in a pot on medium-low heat and whisk thoroughly.

- 7 - Continue cooking for 15 minutes while starting to cook the sweetbreads.

- 8 - Season the tops of the sweetbreads with salt.

- 9 - Heat a cast-iron skillet or nonstick pan to medium-high heat with butter or ghee.

- 10 - Sear for 3 minutes on the tops and bottoms or until browned.

- 11 - Remove from the pan and add the remaining butter or ghee to the gravy pot.

- 12 - Stir gravy while increasing heat to medium-high.

- 13 - Continue whisking vigorously as gravy starts to reduce and thicken.

- 14 - Once the gravy has thickened, plate the sweetbreads and pour gravy over the top.

HALLOUMI FRIES

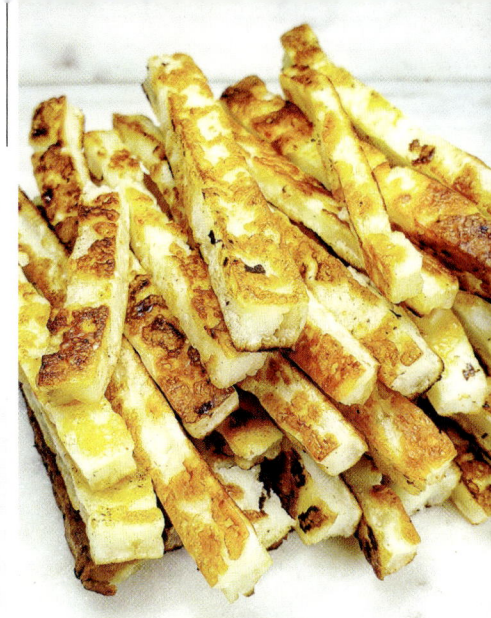

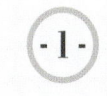  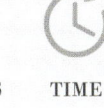

DIFFICULTY
- 1 -

SERVINGS
4

TIME
PREPARATION
15 MINS

COOKING
25 MINS

-PER SERVING-
246 CALORIES
PROTEIN: 16G
CARBS: 1G
FATS: 20G

INGREDIENTS

250 Grams of Halloumi

STEPS

- 1 -   Remove the block of halloumi from its package and pat it dry.
- 2 -   With a knife, slowly slice through the block every ¼ inch.
- 3 -   Then cut each slice again at every ¼ inch creating the fry shape.
- 4 -   Heat a large nonstick pan to a medium low heat.
- 5 -   Once heated, place the halloumi pieces into the pan and cook on all 4 sides until the cheese has browned.
- 6 -   Serve immediately after cooking for the best experience.

The Ultimate Carnivore Cookbook
www.bioptimizedketo.com

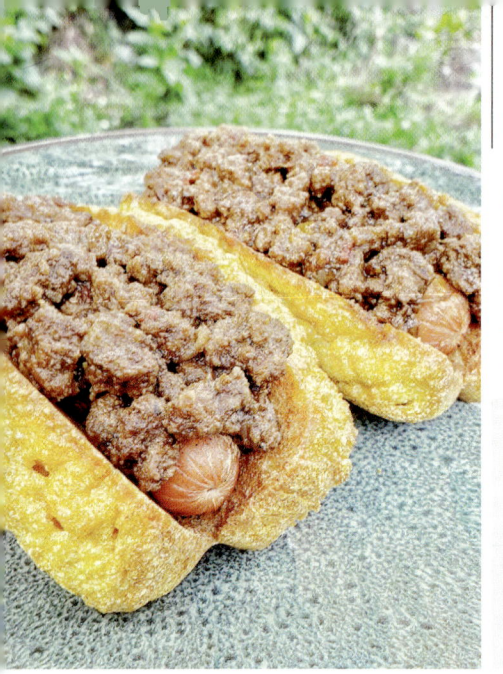

CHILI DOGS ON CARNIVORE BUNS

TIME   **SERVINGS**   **DIFFICULTY**

PREPARATION
45 MINS   4

COOKING
1½ HOUR

-PER SERVING-

756 CALORIES

PROTEIN: 71G
CARBS: 3G
FATS: 51G

- START BY BAKING THE BUNS -

CARNIVORE BUN INGREDIENTS

2 Cups of Pork Panko by Bacon's Heir
30 Grams of Egg Whites
5 Large Eggs
1 Tsp of Redmond Real Salt

STEPS

- 1 -   Start by separating the egg yolks from egg whites into 2 different bowls.

         Note Place the egg whites into a large bowl for whipping.

- 2 -   Add the additional egg whites to the bowl of egg whites.

- 3 -   Whip the egg whites until stiff peaks are formed.

- 4 -   After that, whip the yolks until it forms a smooth custard.

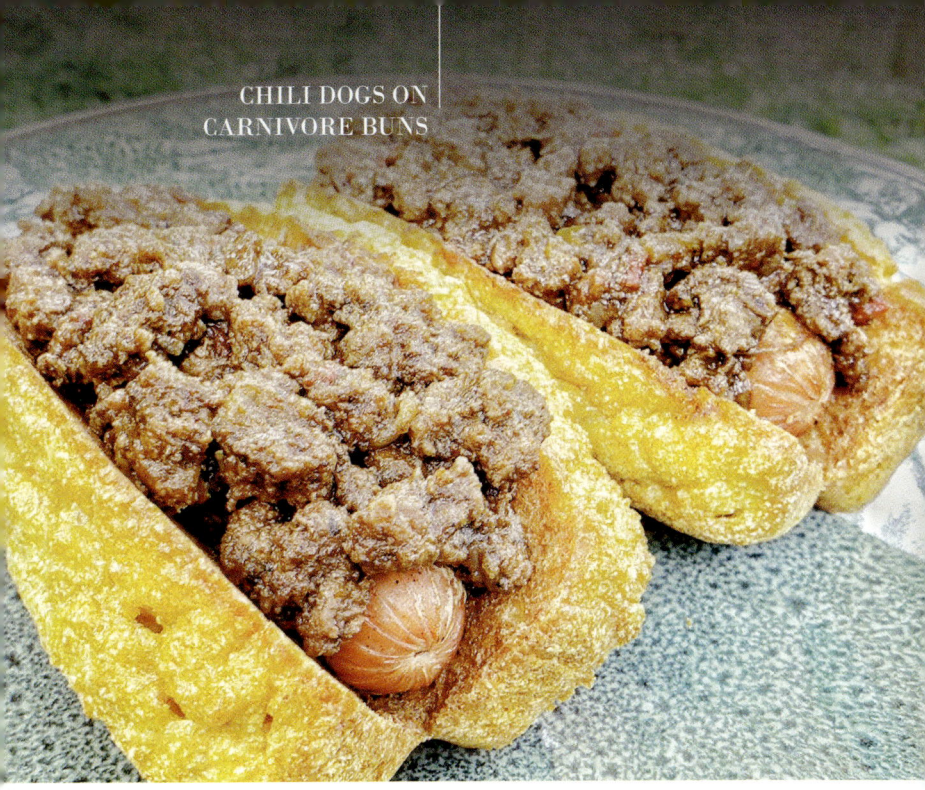

CHILI DOGS ON CARNIVORE BUNS

STEPS

- 5 - Add Pork Panko and salt to the whipped egg whites and mix together.

- 6 - Pour the yolks over the top and mix until everything is fully incorporated.

- 7 - Preheat the oven to 350°F.

- 8 - Scoop batter into 5.75"x3" mini loaf pans and bake for 35 minutes.

- 9 - After cooking, remove from the oven and allow them to cool.

- 10 - Cut in half long-ways.

- 11 - Then slice each half down the middle stopping before going through to the bottom to create the hot dog bun.

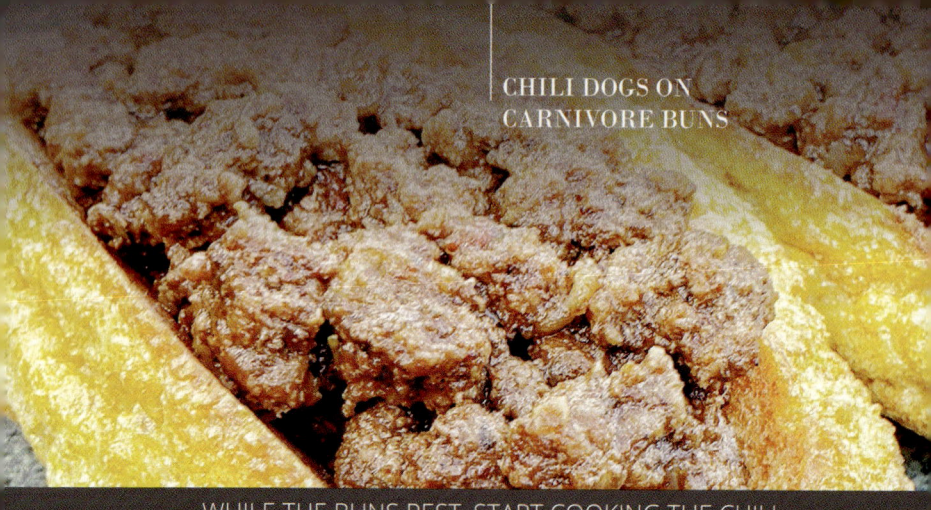

CHILI DOGS ON CARNIVORE BUNS

- WHILE THE BUNS REST, START COOKING THE CHILI -

CHILI INGREDIENTS

1 Lb of Ground Beef (85/15)
2 Cups of Bone Broth* (see recipe)
½ Tbsp of Redmond Real Salt
1½ Tbsp of Ground Cumin
2 Tsp of Chili Powder
1 Tsp of Smoked Chipotle Powder
1 Tsp of Smoked Paprika

STEPS

- 1 - In a deep pot, add the Bone Broth and all of the seasonings.

- 2 - Place the pot on medium heat a stir until the seasonings dissolve into the Bone Broth.

- 3 - Cook for 5 minutes and then crumble in the ground beef.

- 4 - Stir together and cook until the Bone Broth reduces almost completely.

- NOW THAT THE BUNS AND CHILI HAVE BEEN MADE, COOK AND PLACE HOT DOG ONTO THE BUN AND COVER WITH THE CHILI BEFORE SERVING -

PRESSURE COOKER PULLED PORK

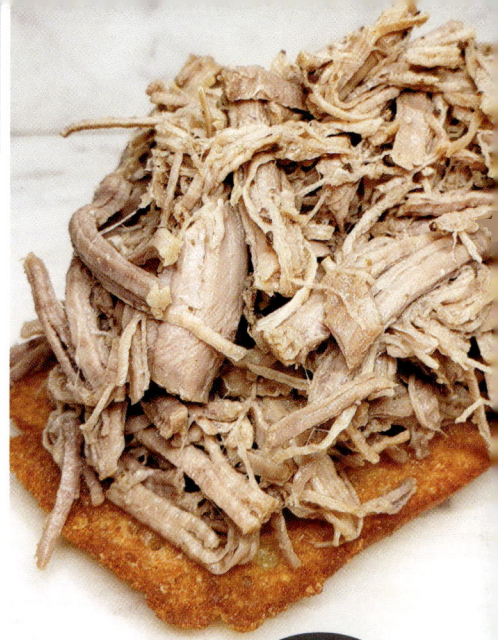

 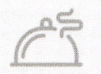 

DIFFICULTY

SERVINGS
6

TIME
PREPARATION
20 MINS
COOKING
3 HOURS

-PER SERVING-

35 CALORIES

PROTEIN: 7G
CARBS: 0G
FATS: 1G

INGREDIENTS

2 Pork Tenderloins (approximately 1½ Lb each)
2 Cups of Bone Broth* (see recipe)
2 Tsp of Redmond Real Salt
2 Tsp of Fresh Cracked Black Pepper

STEPS

- 1 -   Cut the tenderloins into chunks that are 4 inches in length.

- 2 -   Season with salt and pepper.

- 3 -   Place the pork into the pressure cooker and fill with Bone Broth until it nearly covers the tenderloin chunks completely.

- 4 -   Turn the pressure cooker on to high pressure and cook for 2½ hours.

The Ultimate Carnivore Cookbook / 39
www.bioptimizedketo.com

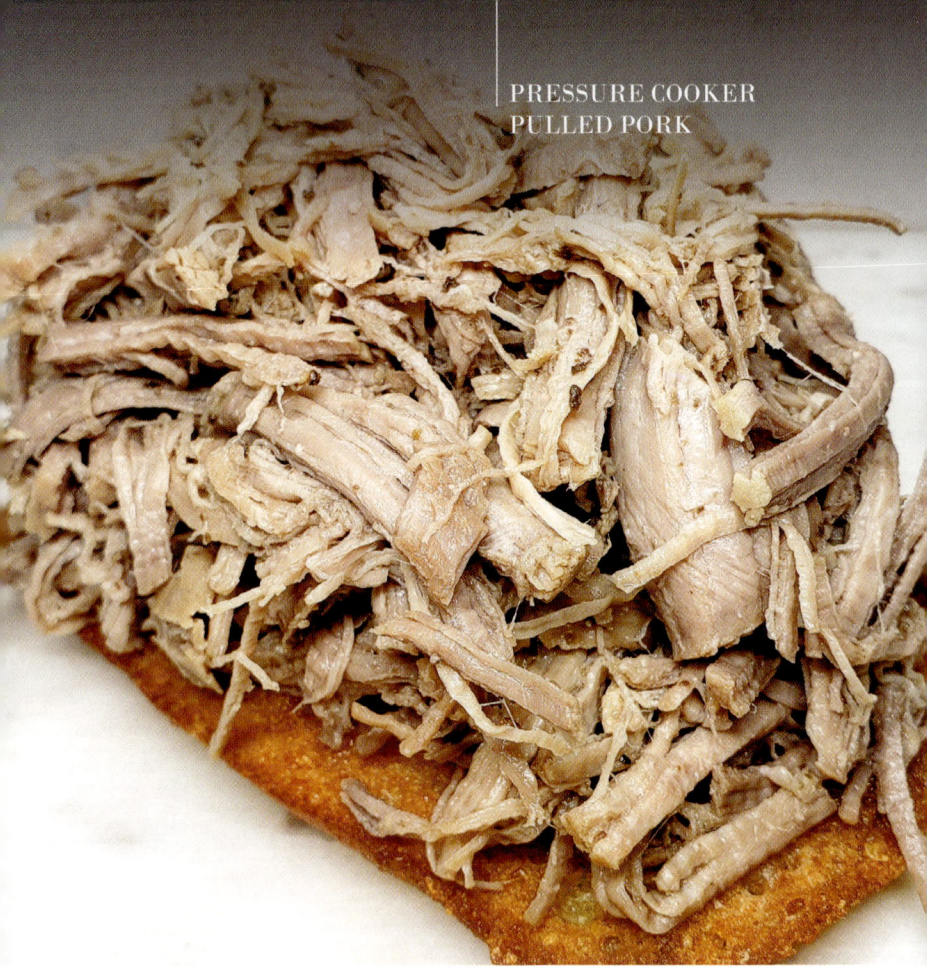

PRESSURE COOKER PULLED PORK

STEPS

- 5 - Turn the power off and let the pork rest inside of the pressure cooker for 30 minutes in the Bone Broth as the cooker cools.

- 6 - Release the pressure and remove the top of the cooker.

- 7 - Shred pork with forks until it has all separated into desired amounts.

TACOS DE LENGUA (BEEF TONGUE TACOS)

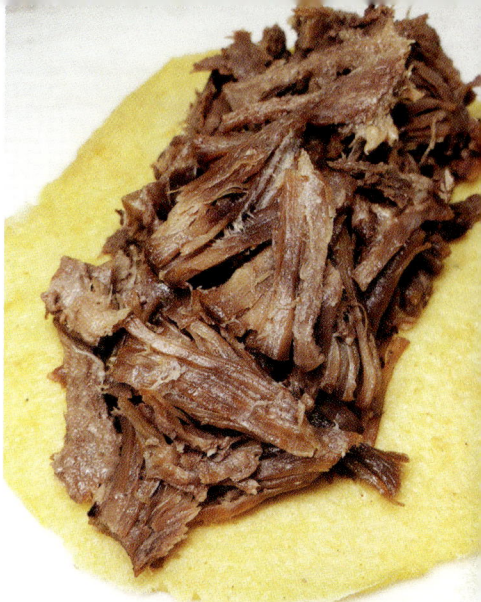

DIFFICULTY

SERVINGS
6

TIME
PREPARATION
20 MINS

COOKING
2 HOURS

-PER SERVING-
519 CALORIES
PROTEIN: 37G
CARBS: 9G
FATS: 37G

INGREDIENTS

1 Whole Beef Tongue (approximately 3 Lbs)
2 Cups of Bone Broth* (see recipe)
2 Tsp of Chili Powder
1½ Tsp of Ground Cumin
1 Tsp of Paprika
⅛ Tsp of Red Pepper Flakes
⅛ Tsp of Onion Powder
⅛ Tsp of Garlic Powder
2 Tsp of Redmond Real Salt
2 Tsp of Freshly Cracked Black Pepper

STEPS

- 1 - Season the underside of the beef tongue with the salt and pepper.

- 2 - Pour the Bone Broth into the pressure cooker and add the rest of the seasonings to it and stir together.

TACOS DE LENGUA (BEEF TONGUE TACOS)

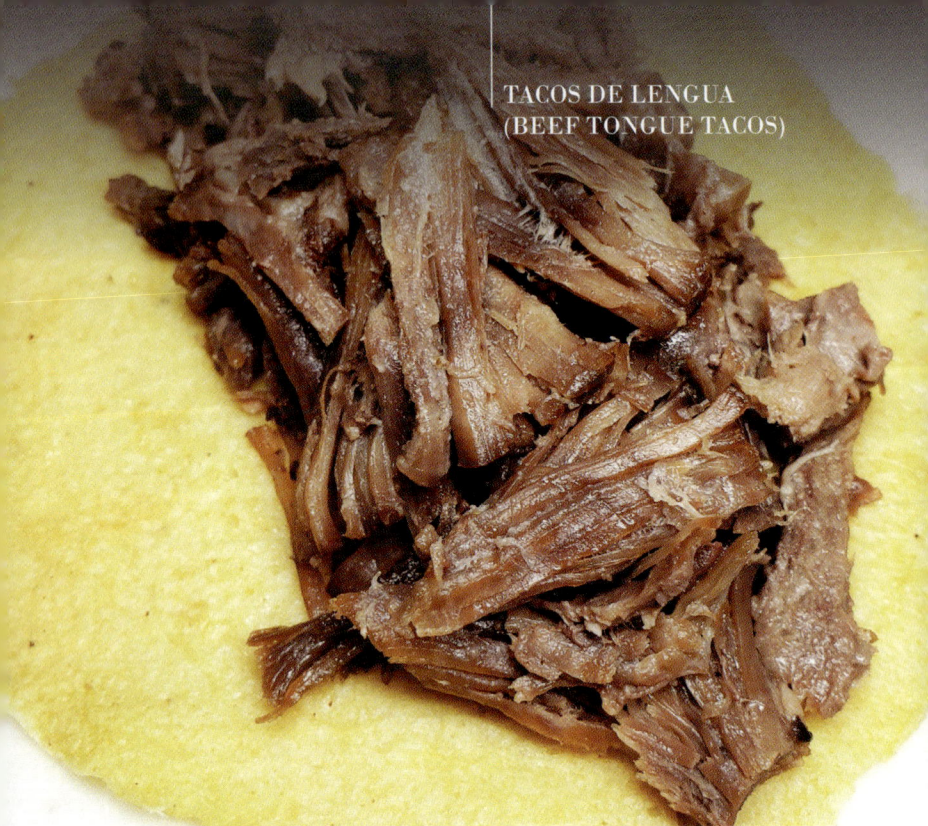

STEPS

Note This leaves the tongue with all the flavor without eating much of the direct seasonings which can be problematic.

- 3 -   Place the whole uncut tongue into the pot.

- 4 -   Turn the pressure cooker on high and cook for 1½ hours.

- 5 -   After cooking let the pressure cooker cool for at least 30 minutes before opening the top.

- 6 -   Remove the tongue from the pot and let rest until it is cool enough to remove the skin.

- 7 -   Shred meat with a fork and then serve on top of Carnivore Tortillas.* (See recipe)

ORGAN POWER SOUP

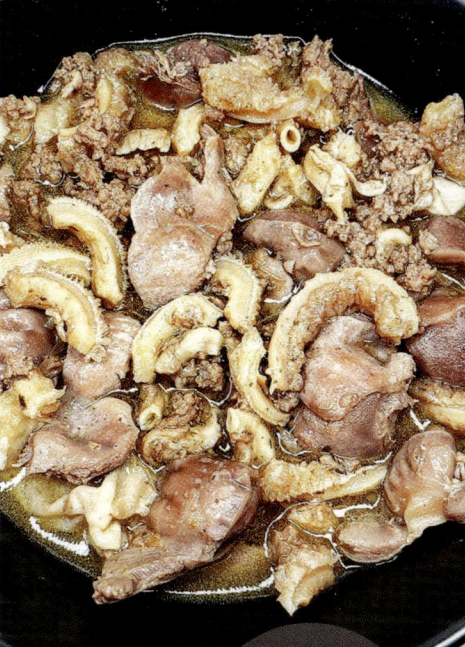

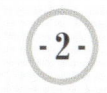 

DIFFICULTY - 2 -

SERVINGS 8

TIME
PREPARATION 35 MINS
COOKING 2 HOURS

-PER SERVING-
320 CALORIES
PROTEIN: 41G
CARBS: 0G
FATS: 17G

INGREDIENTS

1 Lb of Beef Tripe
1 Lb of Ground Beef
1 Lb of Chicken Hearts
1 Lb of Chicken Gizzards
½ Tbsp of Redmond Real Salt
4 Cups of Bone Broth* (see recipe)

STEPS

- 1 -   Begin by rinsing the tripe.

- 2 -   Slicing the tripe into long and thin strips.

- 3 -   Then cut those strips into 3 inch pieces.

- 4 -   Add the Bone Broth and tripe pieces to a large pot and heat to medium high heat.

- 5 -   Add half of the salt and stir in.

The Ultimate Carnivore Cookbook / 43
www.bioptimizedketo.com

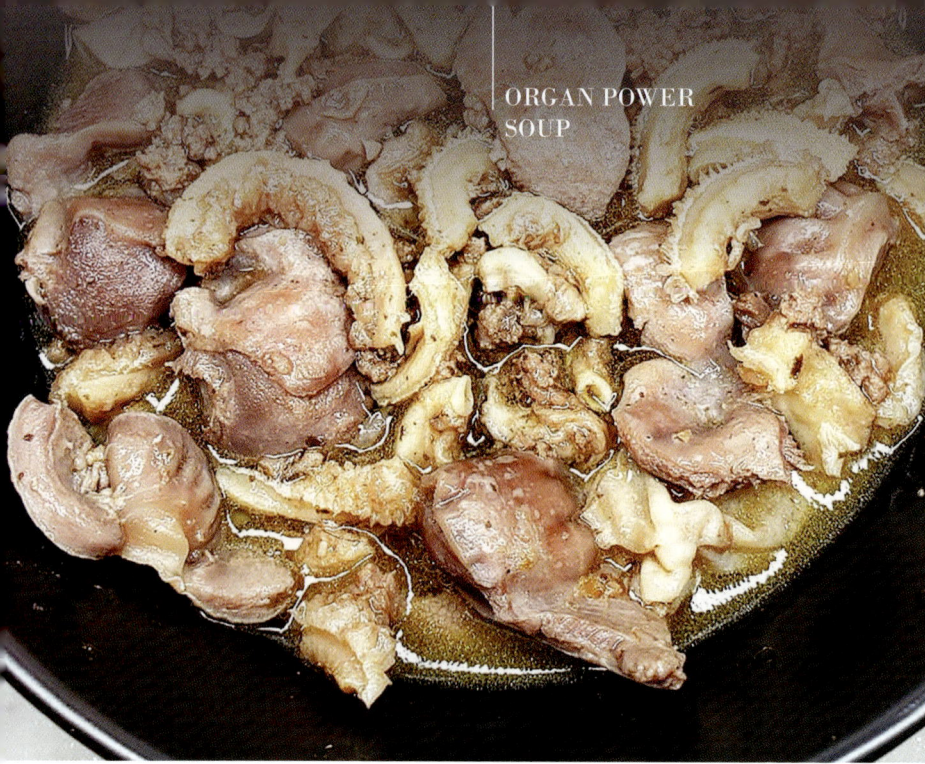

ORGAN POWER SOUP

STEPS

- - 6 -   Cook for 30 minutes.
- - 7 -   Cut the chicken gizzards between the nodes and then add to the pot.
- - 8 -   Cook for another 30 minutes.
- - 9 -   Add the chicken hearts and the rest of the salt to the pot.
- - 10 - Stir everything together and cook down for 20 minutes.
- - 11 - Crumble in the ground beef and turn the heat down to low.
- - 12 - Stir occasionally and let cook for the last 15 minutes before moving off of the burner.
- - 13 - Allow to cool for 10 minutes before serving.

PAN SEARED DUCK BREAST

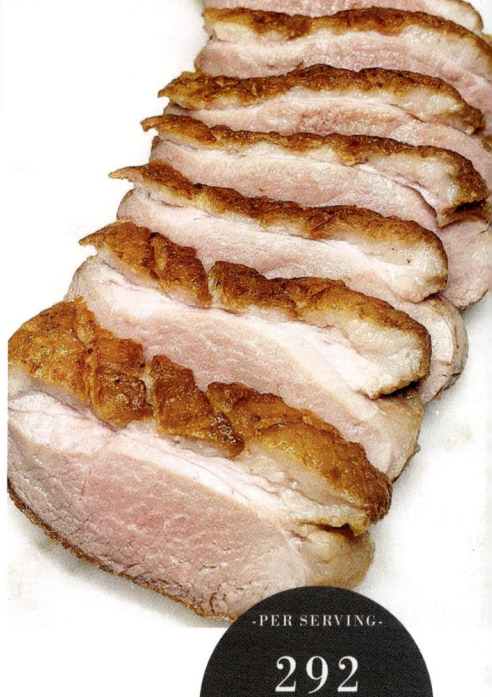

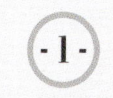
DIFFICULTY
-1-

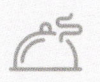
SERVINGS
2

TIME
PREPARATION
10 MINS
COOKING
25 MINS

-PER SERVING-
292 CALORIES
PROTEIN: 29G
CARBS: 0G
FATS: 20G

INGREDIENTS

1 Duck Breast (approximately 1 lb)
1 Tbsp of Fat of Choice
½ Tsp of Redmond Real Salt

STEPS

- 1 - Pat dry the duck breast and then slice the skin diagonally and then again in the inverse direction.

    Note Only cut the very top of the skin. Do not cut through into the meat.

- 2 - Place the duck breast skin side down into a room temperature cast iron skillet or nonstick pan with fat of choice.

- 3 - Place pan or skillet on to the burner and heat to medium-high heat.

- 4 - Cook until the skin begins to crispen.

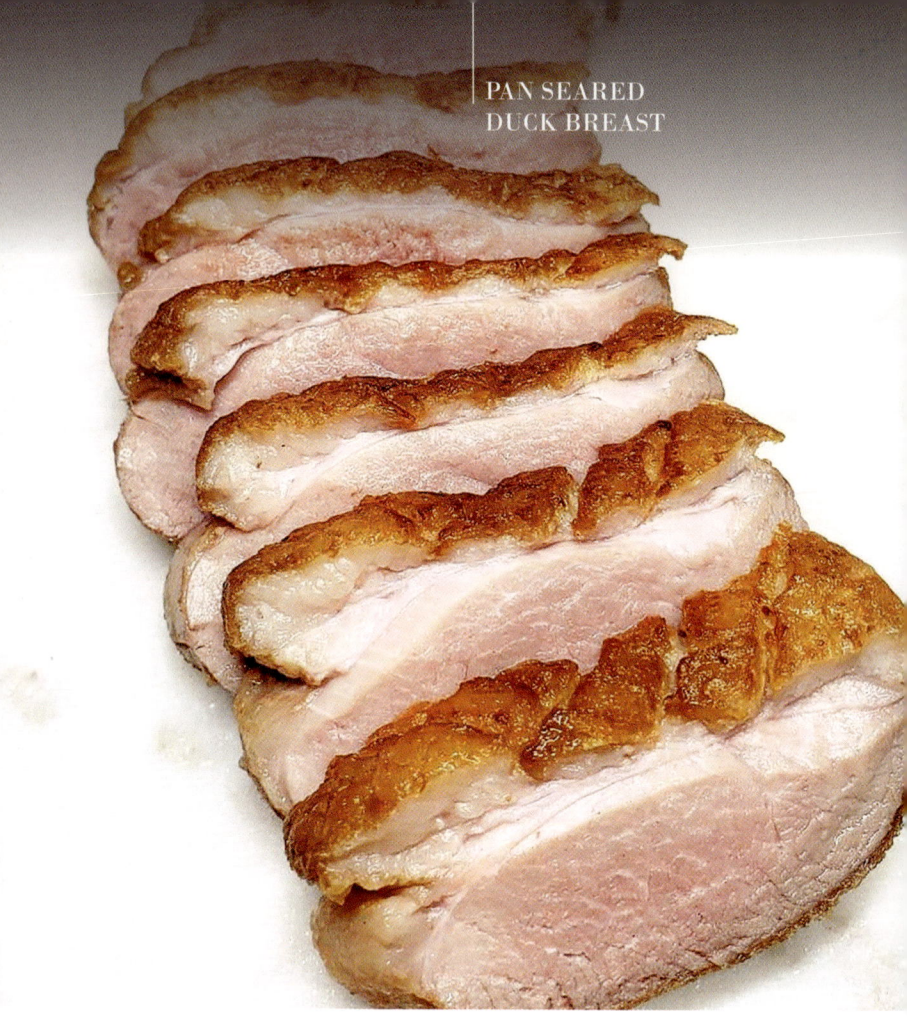

PAN SEARED DUCK BREAST

STEPS

- 5 - Once the skin is brown and crispy, flip over to the meat side and cook for another few minutes.

    Note Duck is best served at a medium-rare to medium cook.

- 6 - After cooking, remove from the pan and slice across the breast horizontally.

PAFFLE PIZZA

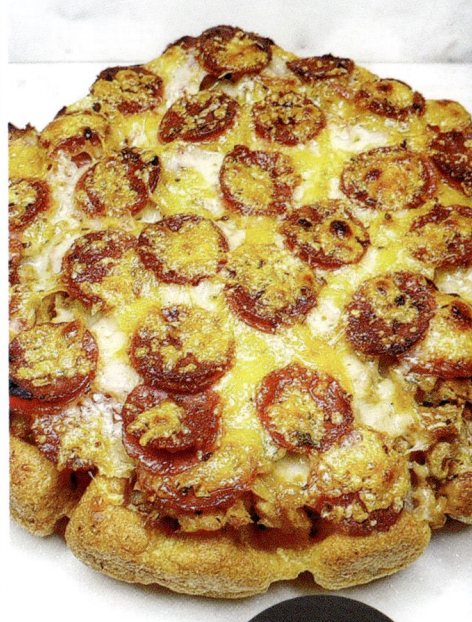

DIFFICULTY - 1 -

SERVINGS 4

TIME
PREPARATION 25 MINS
COOKING 35 MINS

-PER SERVING-
717 CALORIES
PROTEIN: 59G
CARBS: 2G
FATS: 52G

INGREDIENTS

2½ Cups of Pork Panko by Bacon's Heir
3 Eggs
3 Tbsp of Egg Whites
1-2 Tsp of Redmond Real Salt
1 Tsp of Garlic & Herb Seasoning
1 Tsp of Pizza Seasoning
3 Oz of Shredded Cheese
1 4 Oz Pack of Pepperoni

STEPS

- 1 - In a large bowl, mix together all ingredients except for the cheese and pepperoni.

- 2 - Scoop mixture into a waffle iron and cook until browned.

- 3 - Top the paffle with cheese and pepperoni then pop them under the broiler in an oven for 5 minutes or until cheese has melted and pepperonis have crisped.

The Ultimate Carnivore Cookbook / 47
www.bioptimizedketo.com

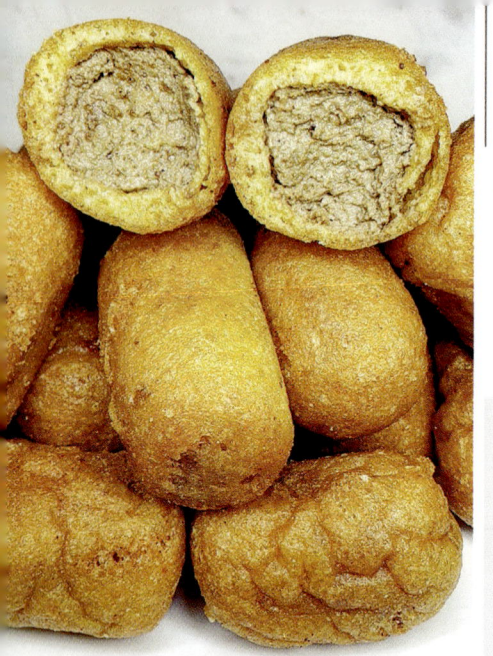

PÂTÉ "CORN" PUFFS

TIME   **SERVINGS**   **DIFFICULTY**

PREPARATION
2½ HOURS

COOKING
40 MINS

8

-PER SERVING-

540 CALORIES

PROTEIN: 38G
CARBS: 2G
FATS: 42G

- BEEF LIVER PÂTÉ RECIPE -

INGREDIENTS

1 Lb of Beef Liver
½ Cup of Melted Fat of Choice
1 Tsp of Redmond Real Salt

STEPS

- 1 - Heat a cast-iron skillet or nonstick pan to medium high heat.

- 2 - Put a ¼ cup of fat and let it heat up.

- 3 - Place the liver into the pan and sear on both sides for 3 minutes or until browned.

- 4 - Remove the liver and place it into a food processor.

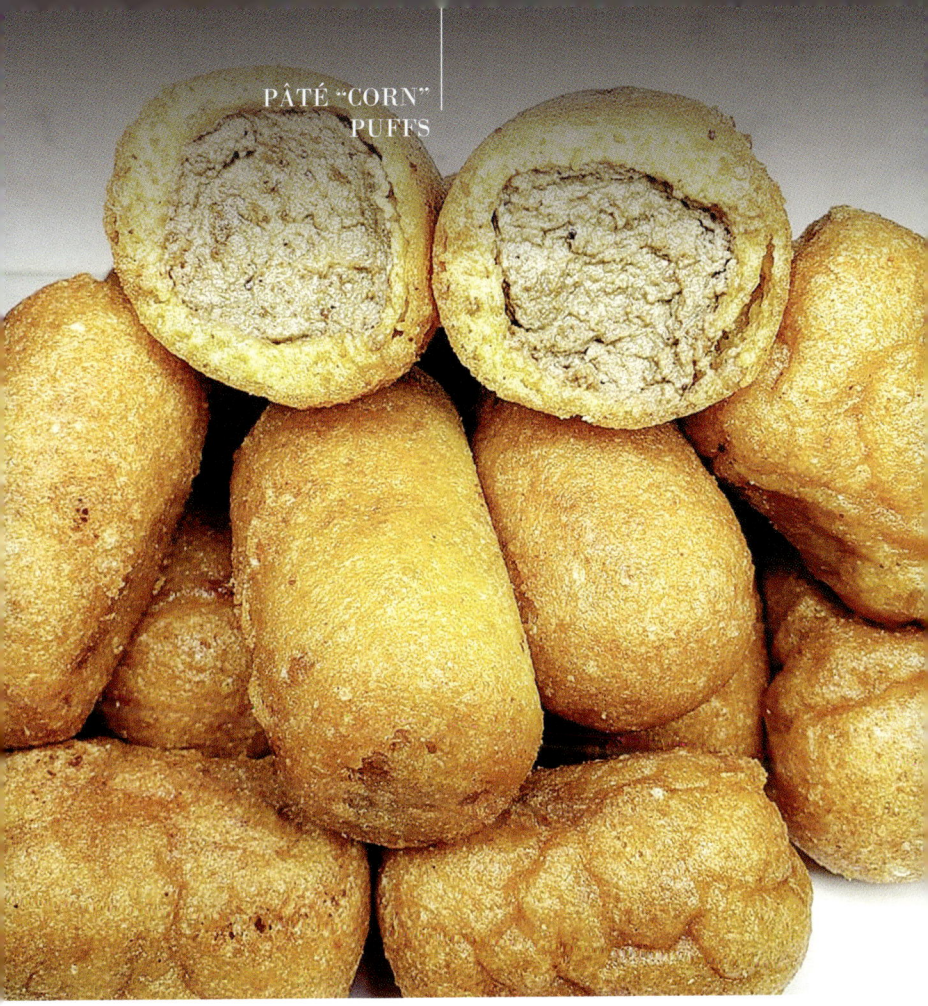

PÂTÉ "CORN" PUFFS

STEPS

- 5 - Pour the melted fat from cooking into the food processor and pulse everything together.

- 6 - Slowly add the other ¼ cup of fat while pulsing until it's at a smooth consistency.

- 7 - Cool inside a refrigerator in a airtight container for at least 2 hours before usage.

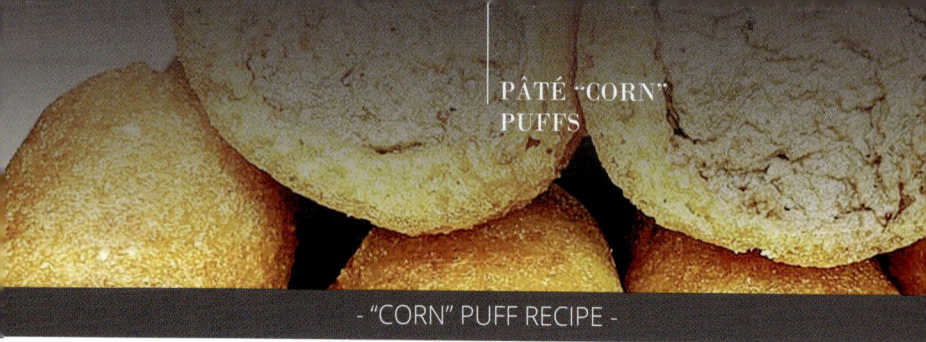

PÂTÉ "CORN" PUFFS

- "CORN" PUFF RECIPE -

INGREDIENTS

2 Cups of Pork Panko by Bacon's Heir
9 Tbsp of Egg Whites
2 Large Eggs
3-4 Cups of Fat of Choice

STEPS

- 1 - Mix all ingredients together in a large mixing bowl.

- 2 - Take the Pâté and mold into 1x2" logs.

- 3 - Wrap the "Corn" Puff mixture around the Pâté and roll on parchment paper sprinkled with water until the "Breading" is an even thickness.

- 4 - Close off the ends with fingers and set to the side.

- 5 - Heat the fat inside of a deep pot on medium-high heat.

- 6 - Once all "Corn" Puffs have been created, place them into the pot.

    Note The number of "Corn" Puffs that can be fried at one time depends on the size of the pot.

- 7 - Immediately after placing Puffs into the pot, roll them around to prevent the "Corn" Puff dough from cracking away or separating.

- 8 - Cook until breading has become golden brown all the way around.

- 9 - Place on a cooling rack until finished cooking.

GRILLED LAMB SWEETBREADS

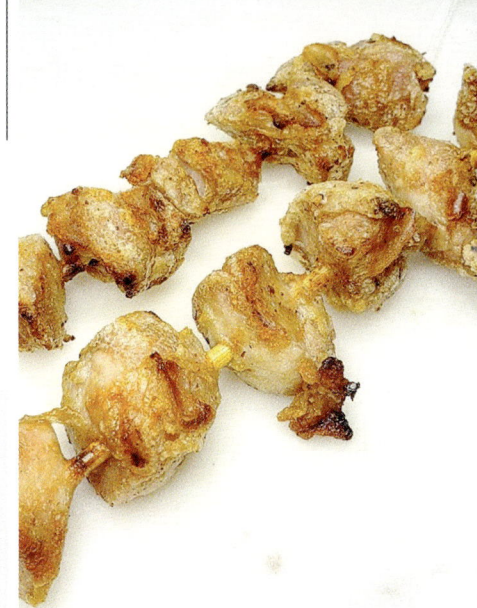

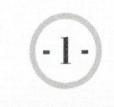  

DIFFICULTY - 1 -

SERVINGS 2

TIME
PREPARATION 10 MINS
COOKING 15 MINS

-PER SERVING-
164 CALORIES
PROTEIN: 25G
CARBS: 0G
FATS: 7G

INGREDIENTS

1 Lb of Lamb Sweetbreads
1-2 Tsp of Redmond Real Salt

STEPS

- 1 - Start by cutting in between the glands of the sweetbreads and setting to the side.

- 2 - Preheat the grill to a medium sized flame or coals.

- 3 - Skewer the sweetbread pieces with at least a ½ inch space between them.

- 4 - Season with the salt on all sides.

- 5 - Place onto the grill for 10 minutes or until they turn to a golden brown with the edges starting to crisp.

The Ultimate Carnivore Cookbook / 51
www.bioptimizedketo.com

GRILLED LAMB SWEETBREADS

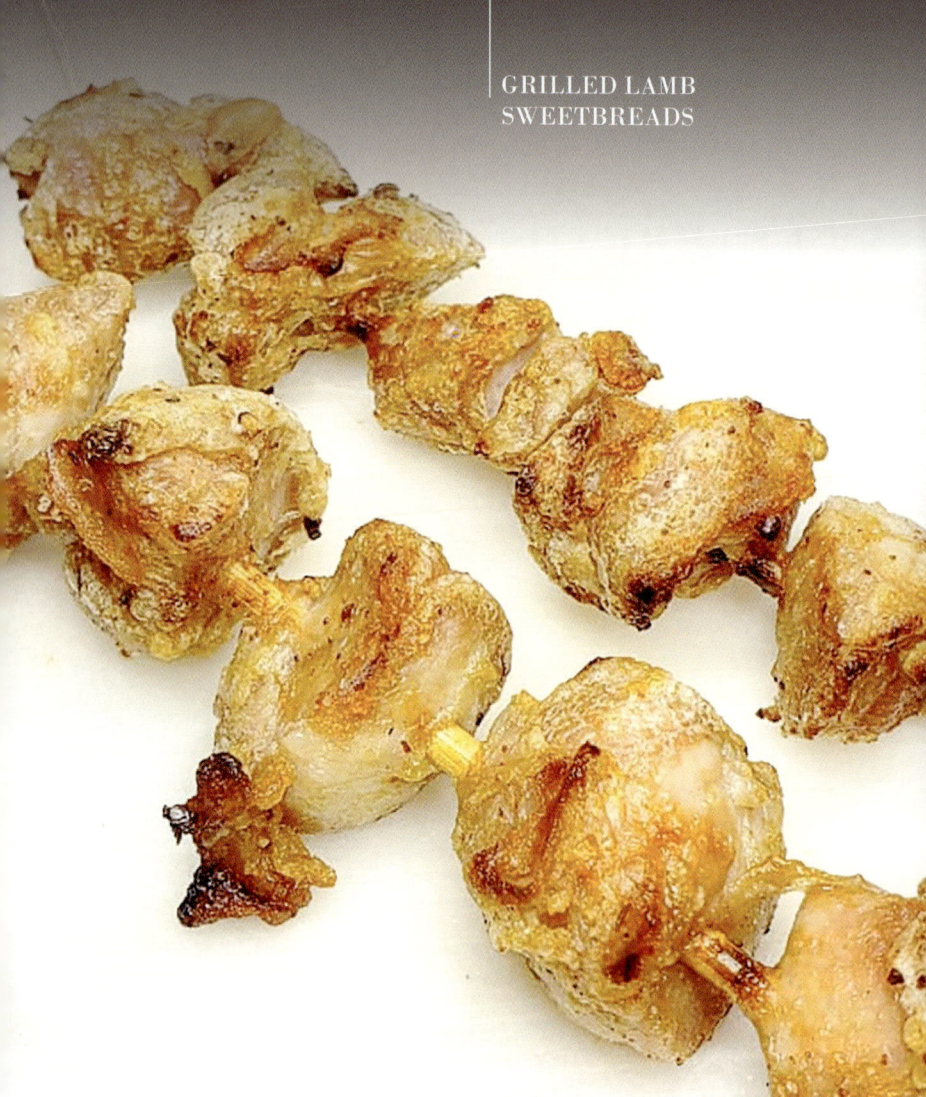

STEPS

- 6 -   Rotate to the other side half of the way through cooking.

Note If using a flame grill, the flame should be a few inches away from the skewers to prevent charring the sweetbreads or the skewer.

SMOKED PORK TENDERLOIN

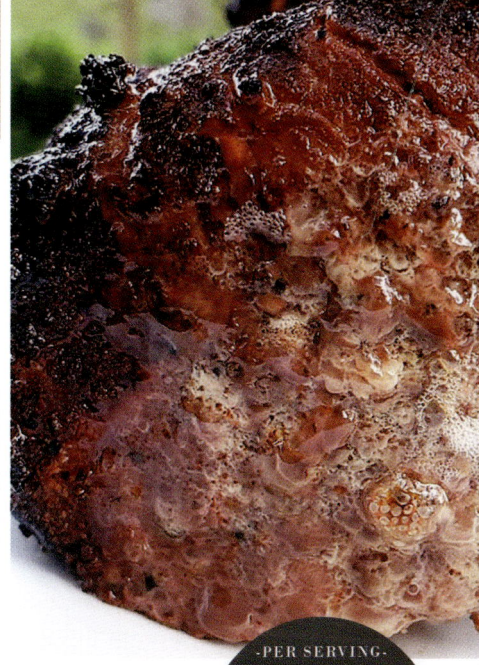

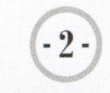 

DIFFICULTY: -2-
SERVINGS: 3
TIME: PREPARATION 20 MINS / COOKING 2½ HOURS

-PER SERVING-
242 CALORIES
PROTEIN: 48G
CARBS: 1G
FATS: 5G

INGREDIENTS

1 Pork Tenderloin (approximately 1½ Lb)
2 Tsp of Paprika
1½ Tsp of Redmond Real Salt
1½ Tsp of Fresh Cracked Black Pepper

STEPS

- 1 - Remove the pork tenderloin from its package and pat it dry.
- 2 - Season all over with paprika and rub it into the meat on all sides.
- 3 - Season with salt and pepper and let rest while starting the smoker.
- 4 - Heat the smoker up to 220°F for ideal results.
- 5 - Once the temperature has been reached, place the tenderloin in, cook until the internal temperature of the pork has reached 155°F.
- 6 - Remove the tenderloin from the smoker and let rest for at least 15 minutes before slicing into it.

The Ultimate Carnivore Cookbook
www.bioptimizedketo.com

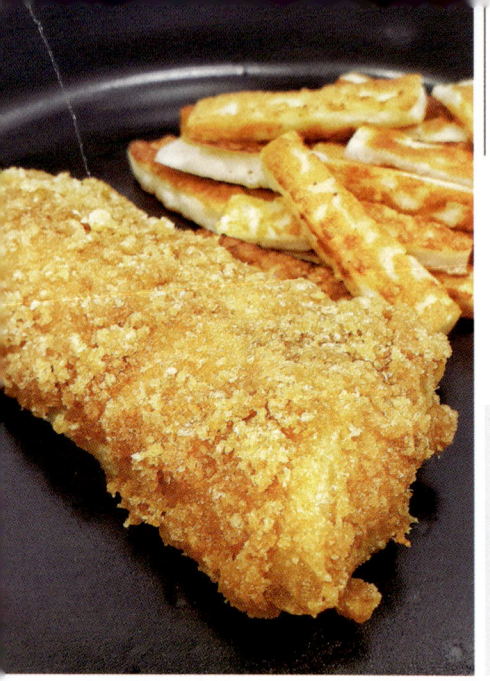

AIR FRIED COD FILLET

TIME
PREPARATION
20 MINS
COOKING
20 MINS

SERVINGS
1

DIFFICULTY

- PER SERVING -
864 CALORIES
PROTEIN: 93G
CARBS: 0G
FATS: 55G

INGREDIENTS

1 Cod Fillet (approximately 90 Grams)
1 Cup of Pork Panko by Bacon's Heir
½ Tsp of Redmond Real Salt

STEPS

- 1 -   Start by putting the Pork Panko into a bowl.

- 2 -   Sprinkle the salt over the top and mix together.

- 3 -   Take the cod and pat the Pork Panko into the fillet on all sides.

- 4 -   Continue until a thick layer has been formed around the cod.

- 5 -   Heat the air fryer to 390°F.

- 6 -   Once it has reached the temperature, place the cod fillet in and cook for 20 minutes.

"CORN" DOGS

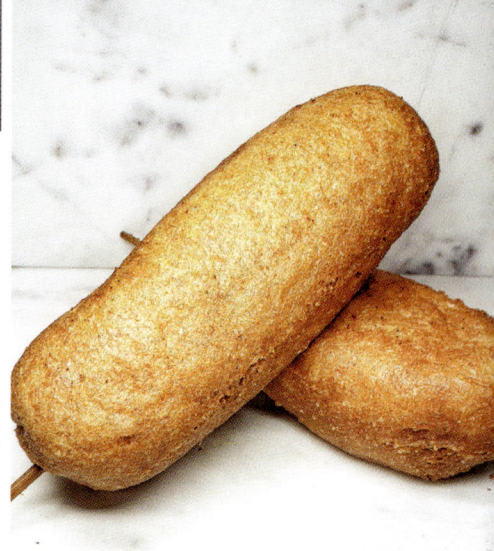

Difficulty	Servings	Time
2	5	Preparation 1 hour / Cooking 30 mins

-PER SERVING-
673 CALORIES
PROTEIN: 40G
CARBS: 2G
FATS: 56G

INGREDIENTS

1 10 Oz Pack of Hot Dogs
2 Cups of Pork Panko by Bacon's Heir
9 Tbsp of Egg Whites
2 Large Eggs
3-4 Cups of Fat of Choice

STEPS

- 1 - Mix ingredients except for the hot dogs in a bowl.

    Note The dough should be tacky but not dry.

- 2 - Skewer your hot dogs and set to the side.

- 3 - Scoop out dough and place evenly around the hot dogs.

    Note It helps if you wet your hands when working the dough.

The Ultimate Carnivore Cookbook / 55
www.bioptimizedketo.com

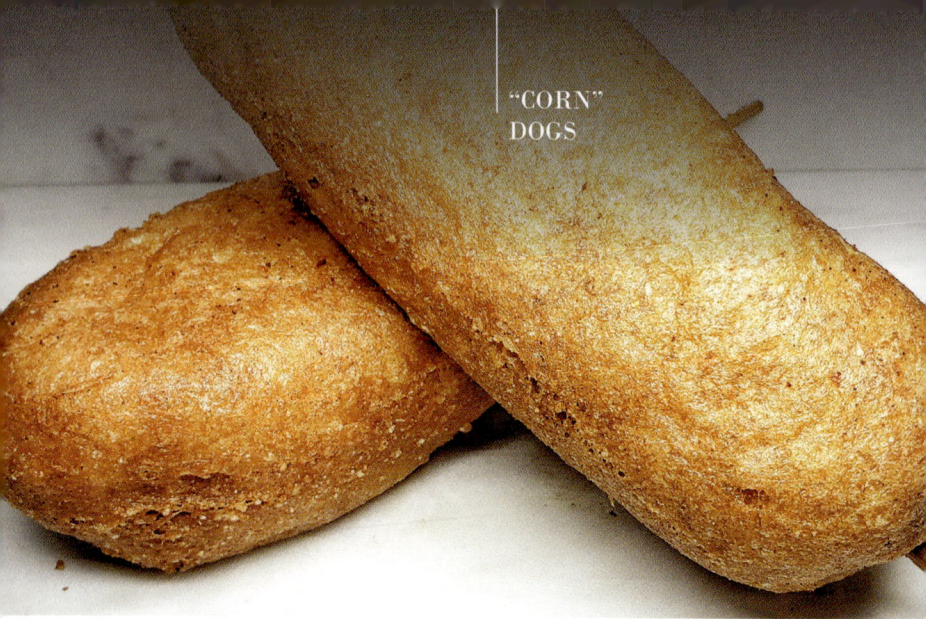

"CORN" DOGS

STEPS

- 4 - Sprinkle water onto a sheet of parchment paper and roll the coated hot dog on the parchment paper to even out the dough.

- 5 - Finish by closing off the ends with and set on a separate sheet of parchment paper.

- 6 - Heat a pot with fat of choice to medium-high heat.

    Note Once melted the fat should be around 4 inches deep.

- 7 - Once heater, place 2 to 3 "Corn" Dogs into the pot at a time.

- 8 - Roll the "Corn" Dogs in the pot after placing them into the fat to prevent the "dough" from splitting or separating from the hot dog.

- 9 - Cook for 5 minutes or until crispy and then roll over the other side.

- 10 - Cook until it has become golden brown and crispy all over.

- 11 - Serve immediately for the best experience.

GARLIC BUTTER PRIME RIB

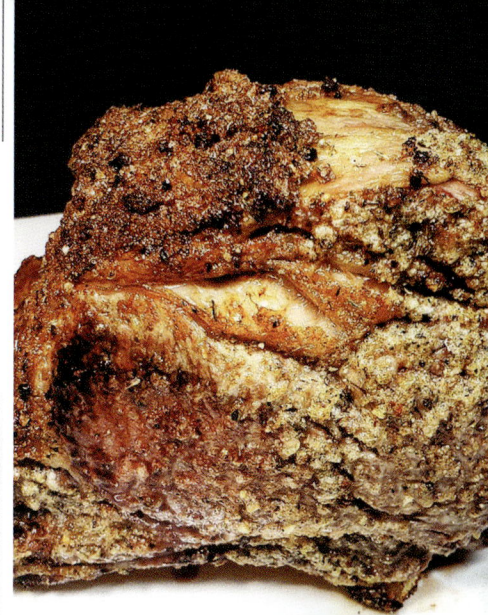

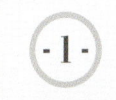 

DIFFICULTY - 1 -

SERVINGS 6

TIME
PREPARATION
25 MINS
COOKING
2 HOURS

- PER SERVING -
1287 CALORIES
PROTEIN: 72G
CARBS: 0G
FATS: 160G

INGREDIENTS

6 Lbs Prime Rib
8 Oz or 20 Tbsp Butter or Ghee
1.5 Tbsp of Redmond Real Salt
1 Tbsp Garlic & Herb Seasoning

STEPS

- 1 - Start by bringing the prime rib and the butter or ghee to room temperature.

- 2 - In a bowl mix together the butter or ghee with the garlic & herb seasoning.

- 3 - Season the prime rib with salt.

- 4 - Using gloved hands, cover the entire prime rib with a layer of the garlic & herb butter/ghee mixture.

The Ultimate Carnivore Cookbook / 57
www.bioptimizedketo.com

GARLIC BUTTER PRIME RIB

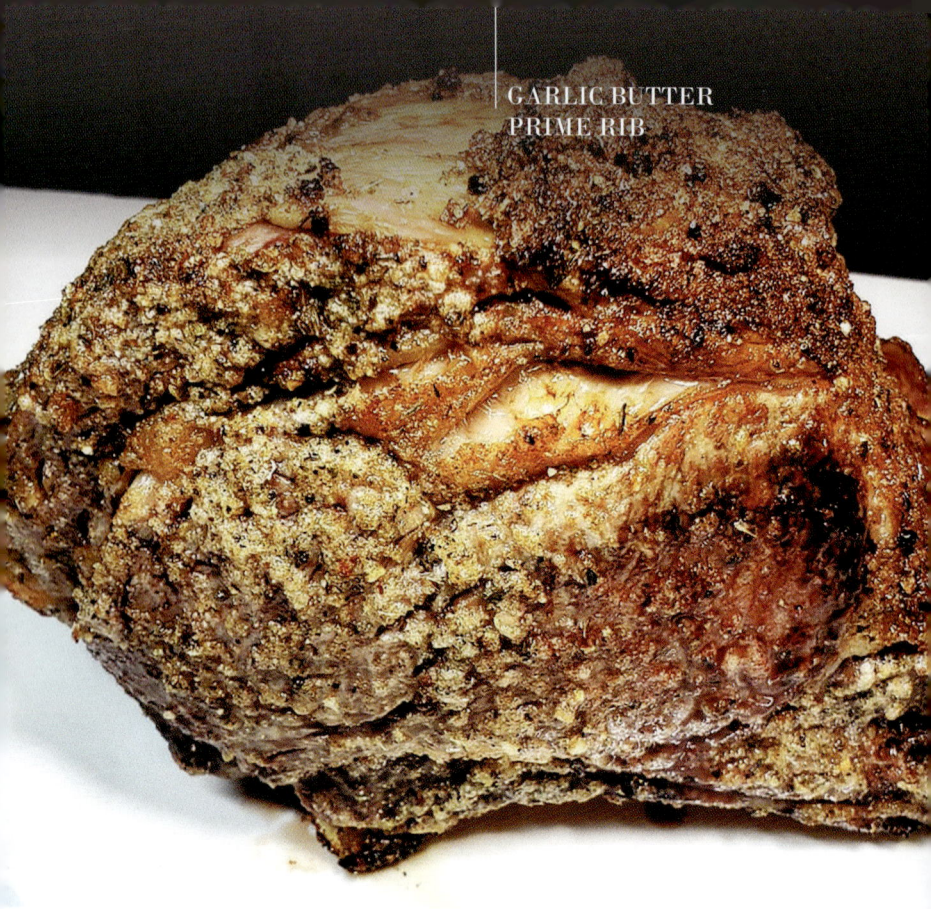

STEPS

- 5 - Preheat the oven to 500°F.

- 6 - Place the prime rib into a deep baking pan.

- 7 - After the oven has reached cooking temperature, put the prime rib pan in for 20 minutes.

- 8 - Once the 20 minutes have passed, turn the oven down to 325°F and finish cooking until the internal temperature has reached 125°F.

- 9 - Let rest for 15 minutes before slicing into the prime rib.

AIR FRIED SHRIMP

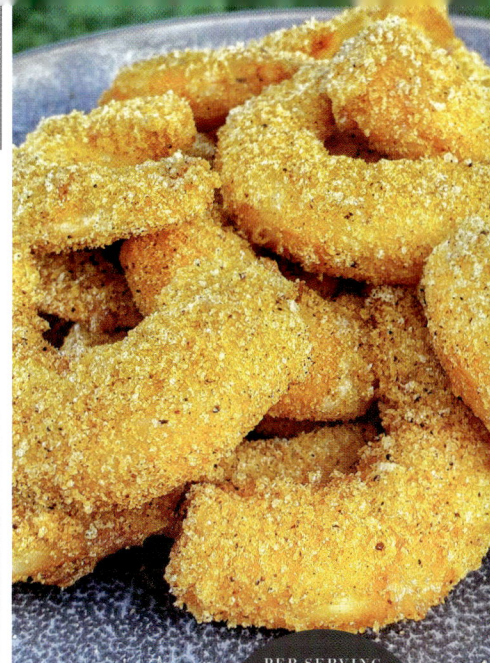

DIFFICULTY

SERVINGS
4

TIME
PREPARATION
20 MINS
COOKING
15 MINS

-PER SERVING-

393 CALORIES

PROTEIN: 50G
CARBS: 0G
FATS: 21G

INGREDIENTS

1 Lb of Peeled Shrimp
1½ Cups of Pork Panko by Bacon's Heir
1½ Tsp of Cajun Season
1 Tsp of Redmond Real Salt

STEPS

- 1 -   In a bowl, mix Pork Panko and the seasonings together.

- 2 -   Place the shrimp into the "breading" bowl one at a time and coat completely.

- 3 -   Repeat this step until all of the shrimp have been "breaded".

- 4 -   Preheat the air fryer to 390°F.

- 5 -   Once the air fryer has reached cooking temperature, gently place the shrimp in and cook for 15 minutes.

- 6 -   Remove and serve immediately.

The Ultimate Carnivore Cookbook / 59
www.bioptimizedketo.com

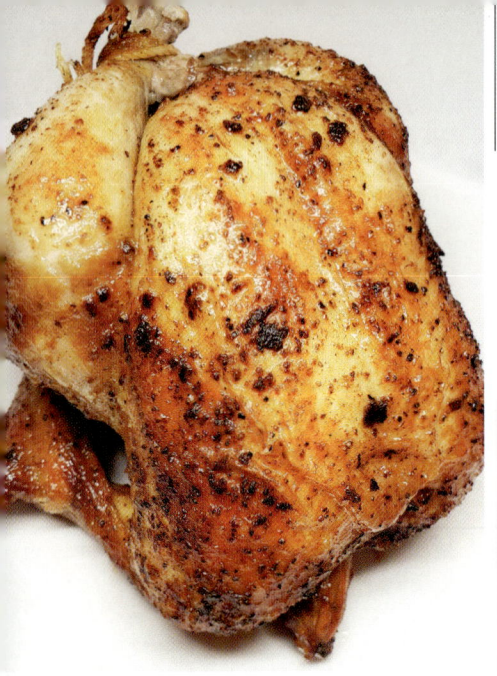

ROASTED CHICKEN

TIME
PREPARATION
15 MINS
COOKING
45 MINS

SERVINGS
4

DIFFICULTY

-PER SERVING-

466 CALORIES

PROTEIN: 41G
CARBS: 1G
FATS: 33G

INGREDIENTS

1 Whole Chicken (approximately 5 Lbs)
¼ Cup Melted Duck or Chicken Fat
1½ Tsp Paprika
1½ Tsp of Redmond Real Salt
½ Tsp of Fresh Cracked Black Pepper

STEPS

- 1 - Let the chicken sit on the counter and warm up to room temperature.

- 2 - Once it has reached room temperature remove the chicken from its package.

- 3 - Using cooking twine, tie the legs together and tie the wings around the back of the chicken exposing the chest.

- 4 - Preheat the oven to 450°F.

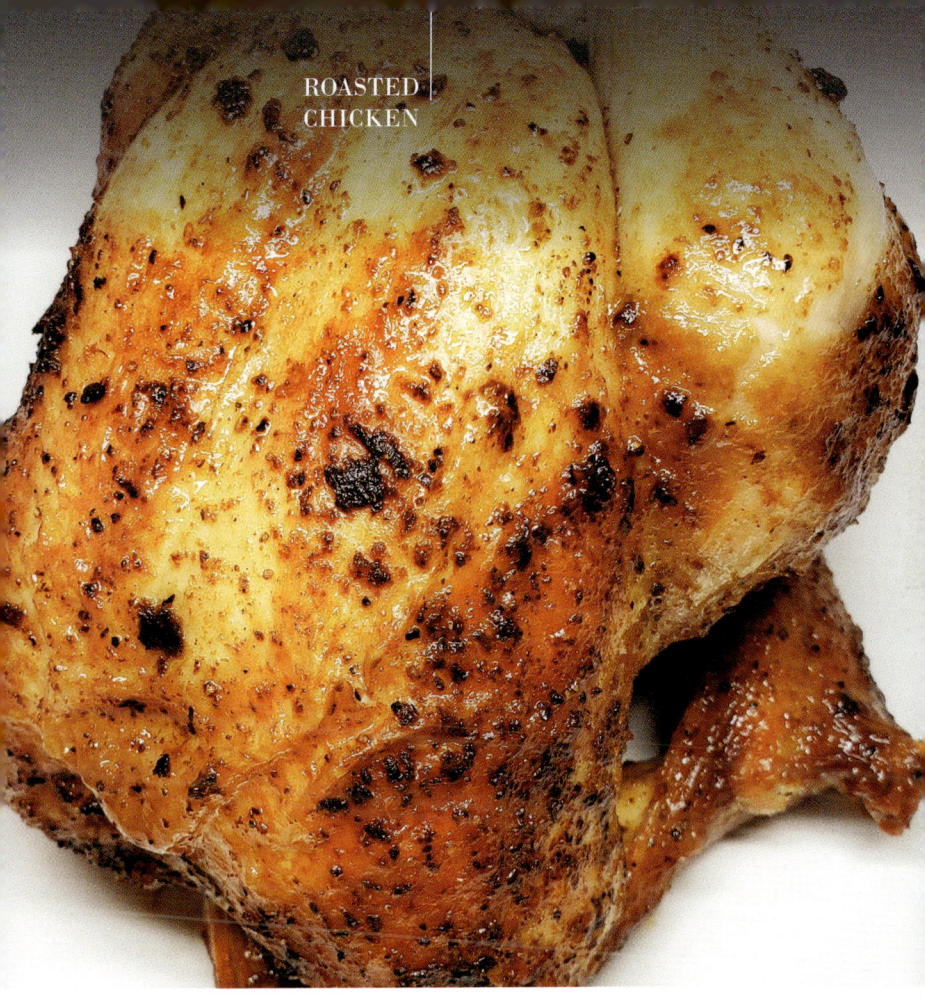

ROASTED CHICKEN

STEPS

- 5 -   Season the whole chicken with paprika rubbing it in.

- 6 -   Then season evenly with salt and pepper.

- 7 -   Place into a baking dish lined with aluminum foil and put into the oven.

- 8 -   Cook for 45 minutes or until the internal temperature reaches 170°F.

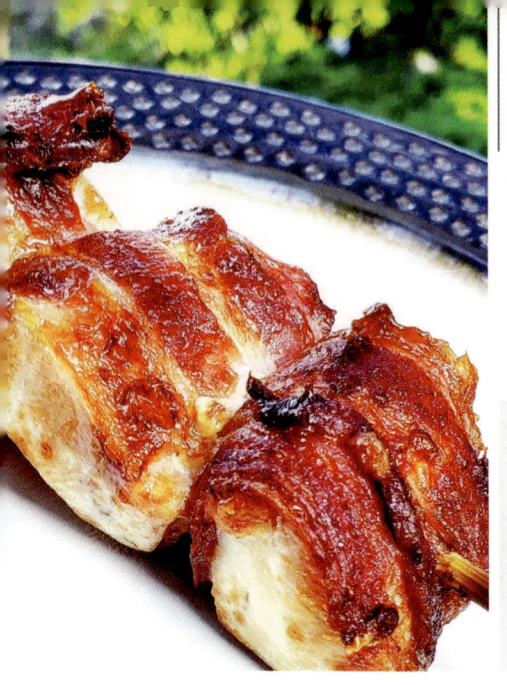

BACON WRAPPED CHICKEN SKEWERS

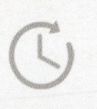

TIME
PREPARATION
25 MINS
COOKING
20 MINS

SERVINGS
2

DIFFICULTY
-1-

-PER SERVING-
699 CALORIES
PROTEIN: 67G
CARBS: 0G
FATS: 48G

INGREDIENTS

1 Lb of Chicken Breast
1 8 Oz Pack of Sugar-Free Bacon
1 Tsp of Redmond Real Salt

STEPS

- 1 - Cut the chicken breasts into 2x2 inch cubes.

- 2 - Season the chicken breast cubes all over with the salt.

- 3 - Cut each strip of bacon into 3 even pieces.

- 4 - Wrap a piece of bacon around the chicken and skewer it.

- 5 - Push chicken cubes together on the skewer.

- 6 - Heat grill to 350°F.

BACON WRAPPED CHICKEN SKEWERS

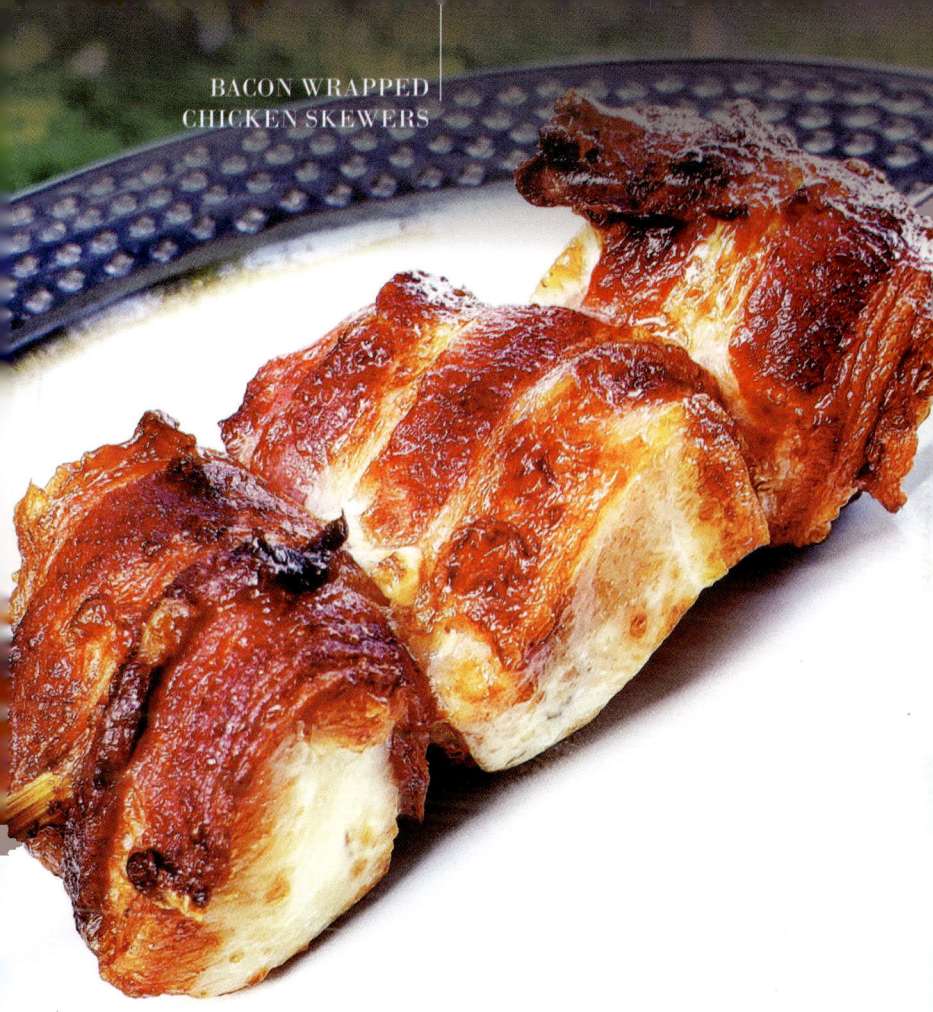

STEPS

- 7 -   Once heated, place the skewers on to the grill and cook for 10 minutes on each side.

- 8 -   Serve immediately after pulling from the grill.

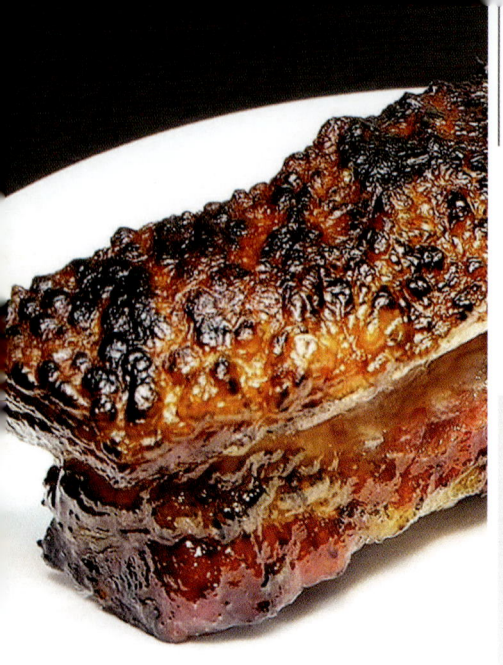

SMOKED PORK BELLY

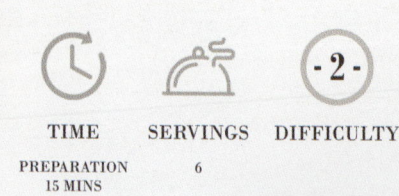

TIME
PREPARATION
15 MINS
COOKING
2 HOURS

SERVINGS
6

DIFFICULTY
- 2 -

- PER SERVING -
1166 CALORIES
PROTEIN: 21G
CARBS: 0G
FATS: 120G

INGREDIENTS

3 Lbs Slab of Pork Belly
1 Tsp of Redmond Real Salt

STEPS

- 1 - Bring pork belly up to room temperature.

- 2 - Heat smoker to 220°F.

- 3 - Cut pork belly into strips that are 2 inches wide.

- 4 - Season the tops and sides lightly with salt.

- 5 - Place into the smoker with 3 inches between each strip.

- 6 - Smoke until the internal temperature reaches 165°F.

GARLIC PARMESAN DRUMSTICKS

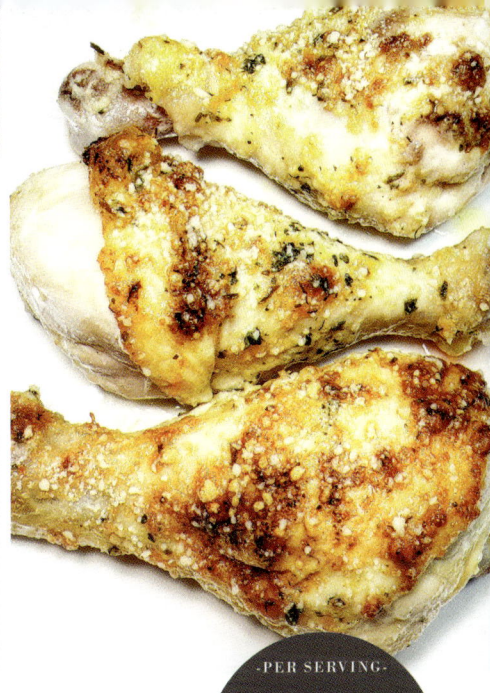

DIFFICULTY: 1
SERVINGS: 2
TIME:
PREPARATION 25 MINS
COOKING 35 MINS

-PER SERVING-
712 CALORIES
PROTEIN: 67G
CARBS: 0G
FATS: 49G

INGREDIENTS

1 Lb of Chicken Drumsticks
1½ Tsp of Garlic & Herb Seasoning
½ Tsp of Redmond Real Salt
½ Cup of Cheese Butter* (see recipe)
3 Oz of Freshly Grated Parmesan Cheese
2 Tsp of Melted Butter

STEPS

- 1 - Pat dry the drumsticks.

- 2 - Preheat the oven to 450°F.

- 3 - Coat the drumsticks in the Cheese Butter and sprinkle seasonings on the top.

The Ultimate Carnivore Cookbook / 65
www.bioptimizedketo.com

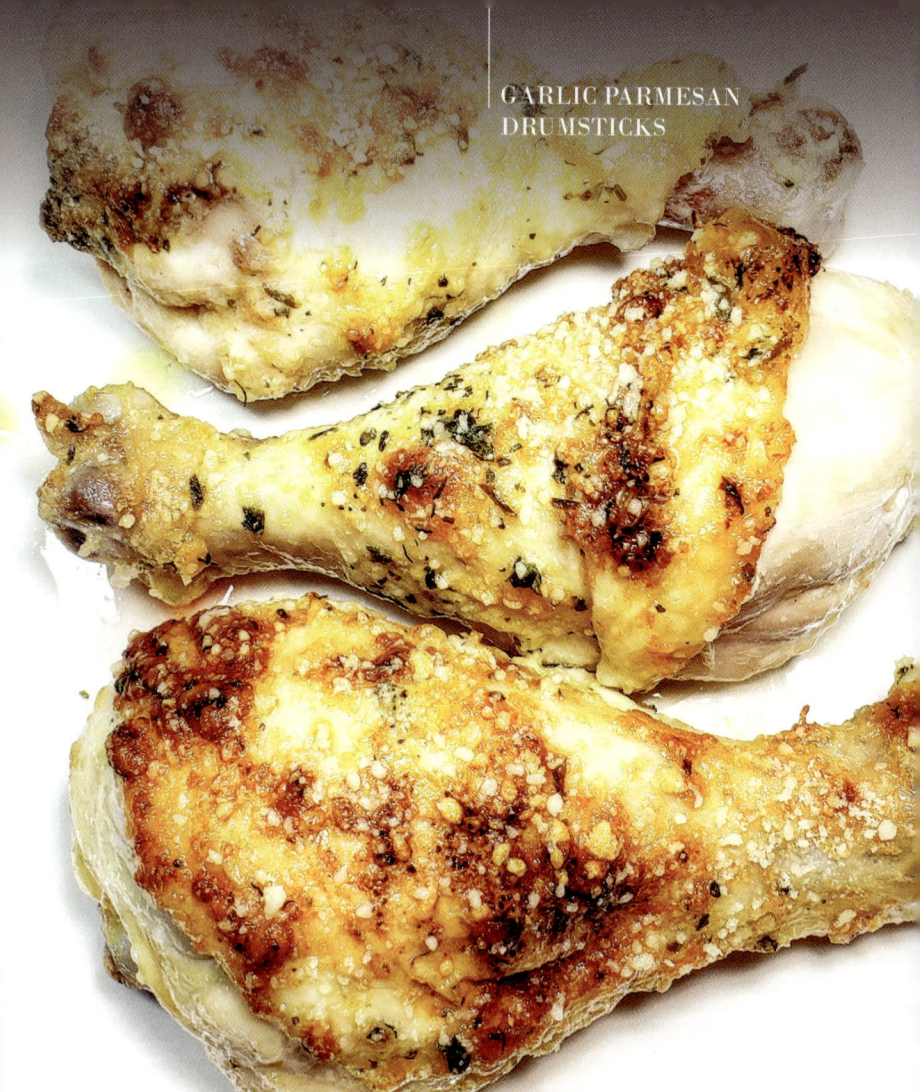

GARLIC PARMESAN DRUMSTICKS

STEPS

- 4 -   Place the drumsticks on a baking sheet lined with aluminum foil and cook in the oven for 35 minutes.

- 5 -   After cooking, drizzle the melted butter over the drumsticks and grate the parmesan cheese on top.

MOLLEJAS TACO

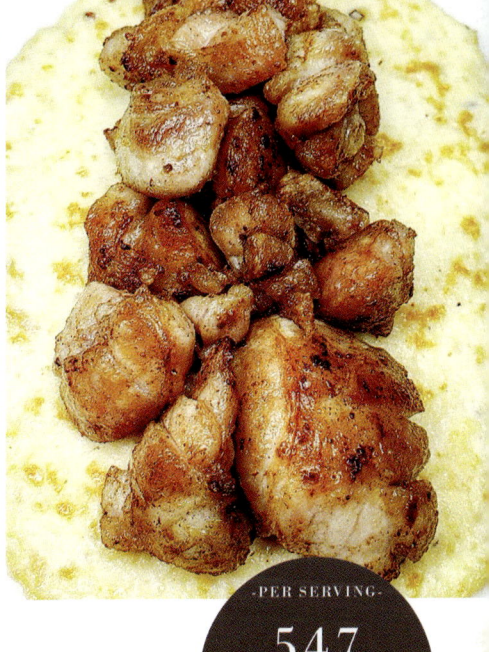

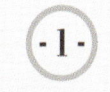

DIFFICULTY · 1 ·

SERVINGS 2

TIME
PREPARATION 10 MINS
COOKING 25 MINS

-PER SERVING-
547 CALORIES
PROTEIN: 65G
CARBS: 0G
FATS: 32G

INGREDIENTS

1 Lb of Beef Sweetbreads
1 Tbsp of Butter or Ghee
1 Tsp of Redmond Real Salt
¼ Tsp of Ground Cumin

STEPS

- 1 - In a pot of water, add salt and bring to a rolling boil.

- 2 - Place whole sweetbreads into the water and boil for 5 minutes.

- 3 - Remove sweetbreads from the pot and set onto a cutting board.

- 4 - Cut the sweetbreads between the glands.

- 5 - Heat a cast iron skillet or nonstick pan to medium-high heat with the butter or ghee.

The Ultimate Carnivore Cookbook
www.bioptimizedketo.com

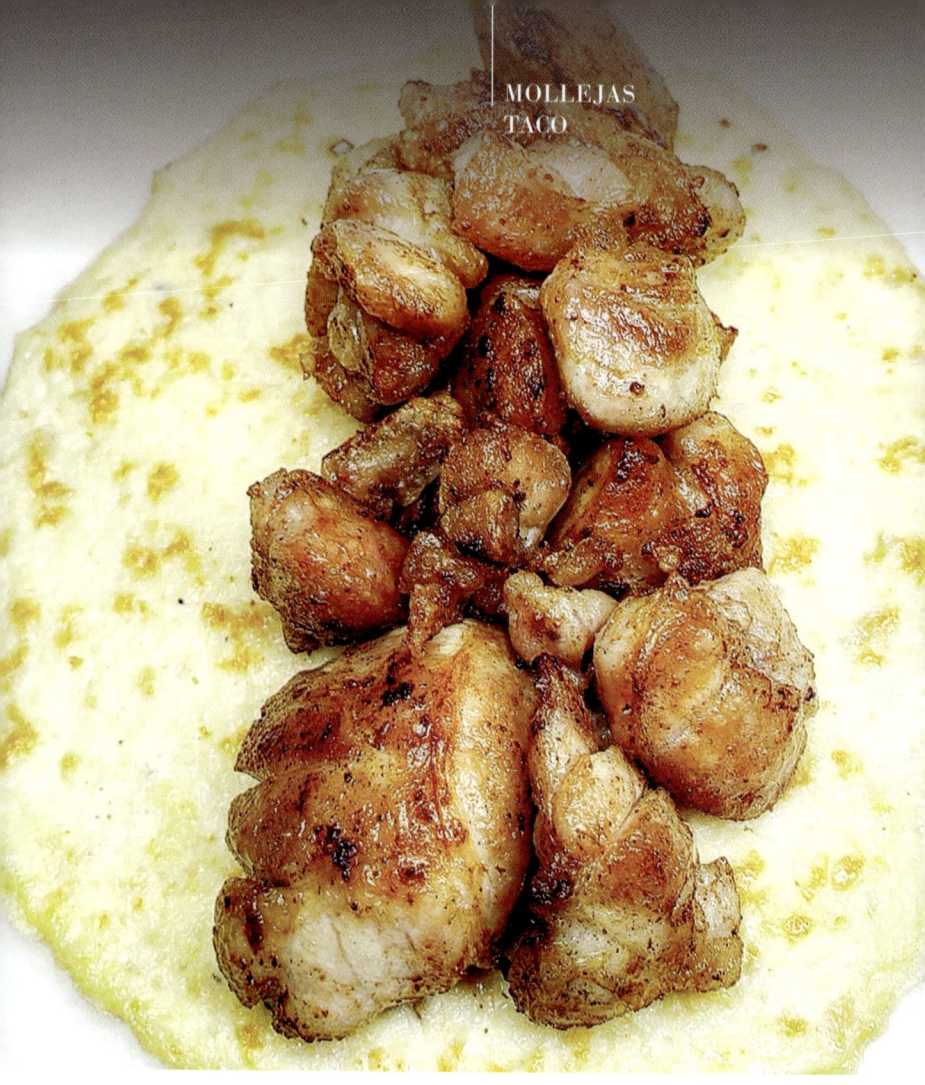

MOLLEJAS TACO

STEPS

- 6 - Place the sweetbreads to the pan and add the cumin in and stir together.

- 7 - Cook until the bottoms have turned to a golden brown on all sides.

- 8 - Remove from the pan and place on Carnivore Tortillas.*

DAIRY-FREE CHICKEN PIZZA CRUST

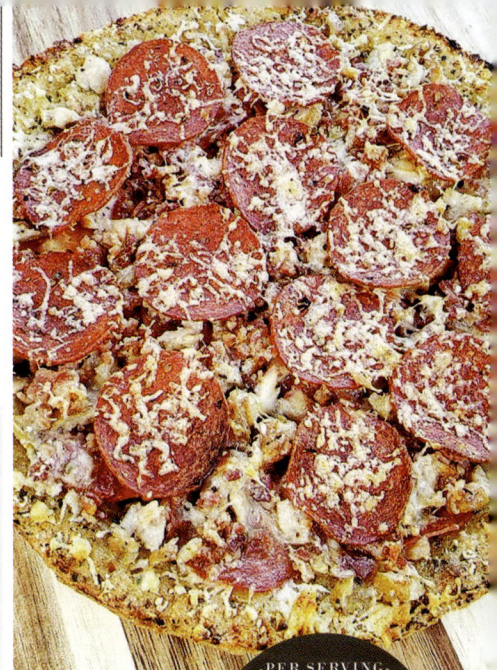

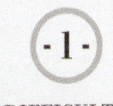  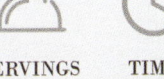

DIFFICULTY: 1
SERVINGS: 4
TIME: PREPARATION 25 MINS / COOKING 25 MINS

- PER SERVING -
487 CALORIES
PROTEIN: 50G
CARBS: 0G
FATS: 32G

INGREDIENTS

1½ Cups of Pork Panko by Bacon's Heir
1 Lb of Ground Chicken
2 Large Eggs
2 Tsp of Redmond Real Salt
2 Tsp of Garlic & Herb Seasoning

STEPS

- 1 - In a large bowl add all ingredients and mix thoroughly.

- 2 - Add mixture to a 9" cake pan.

- 3 - Preheat the oven to 400°F.

- 4 - Pack dough in and create a thicker part around the rim to give it a traditional crust look.

The Ultimate Carnivore Cookbook / 69
www.bioptimizedketo.com

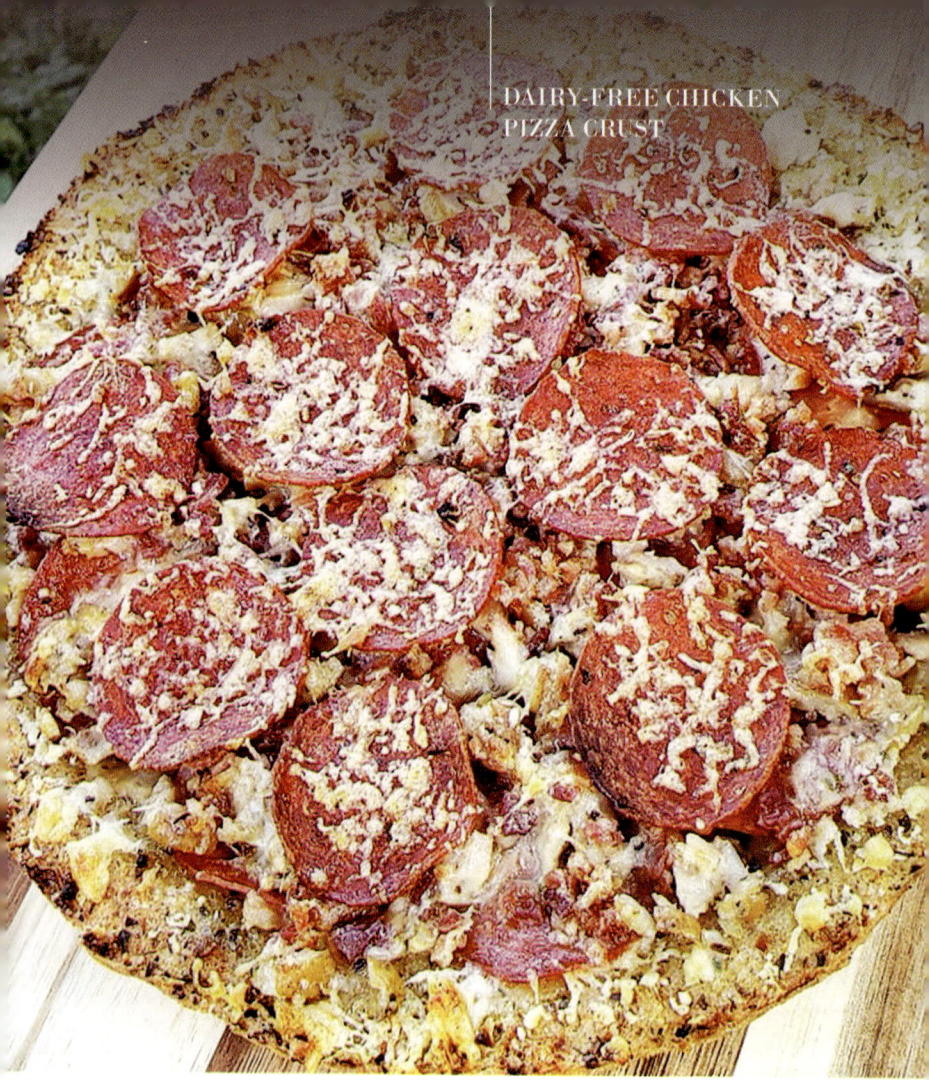

DAIRY-FREE CHICKEN PIZZA CRUST

STEPS

- 5 - Bake the crust for 25 minutes.

   Note The crust will inflate. Push the air out before topping.

- 6 - Top with desired toppings and cheeses before placing back into the oven for 5 minutes or until the cheese has melted.

PARMESAN PORK

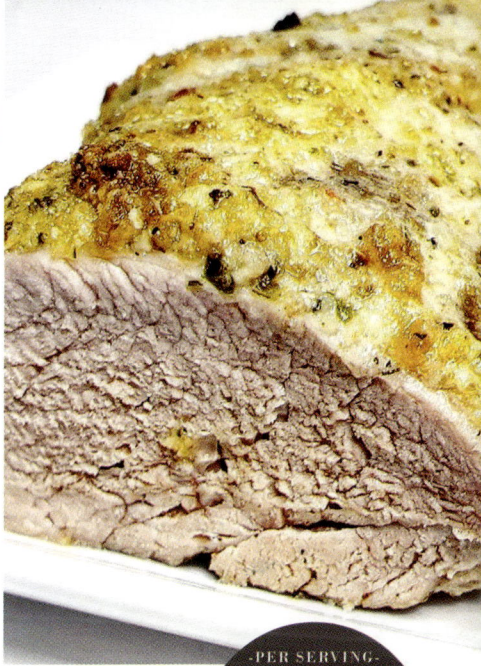

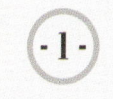
DIFFICULTY
· 1 ·

SERVINGS
4

TIME
PREPARATION
20 MINS
COOKING
35 MINS

-PER SERVING-
629 CALORIES
PROTEIN: 53G
CARBS: 4G
FATS: 44G

INGREDIENTS

1 ½ Lbs Pork Tenderloin
¼ Cup of Pork Panko by Bacon's Heir
4 Oz of Parmesan Cheese
½ Cup of Melted Garlic Ghee* (see recipe)
½ Tsp of Redmond Real Salt
⅛ Tsp of Oregano
⅛ Tsp of Thyme
⅛ Tsp of Black Pepper

STEPS

- 1 -   Start by pat drying the pork tenderloin
- 2 -   In a bowl, mix together the Pork Panko, parmesan, and seasonings.
- 3 -   Place the pork tenderloin on a baking sheet lined with aluminum foil.
- 4 -   Preheat the oven to 375°F.

The Ultimate Carnivore Cookbook / 71
www.bioptimizedketo.com

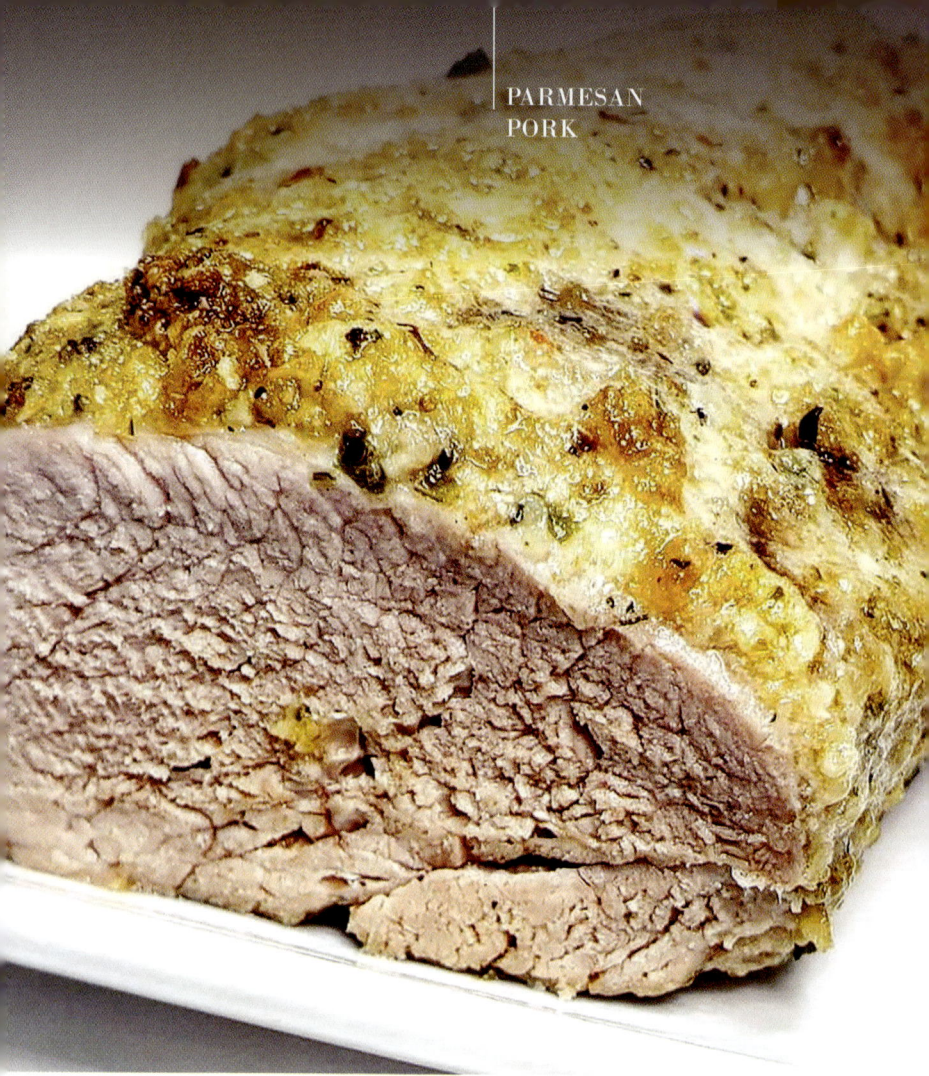

PARMESAN PORK

STEPS

- 5 -   Baste the pork with the Garlic Ghee.

- 6 -   Roll the pork in the cheese & Pork Panko mixture until coated all over.

- 7 -   Place into the oven and cook for 35 minutes.

AIR FRIED CHICKEN TENDERS

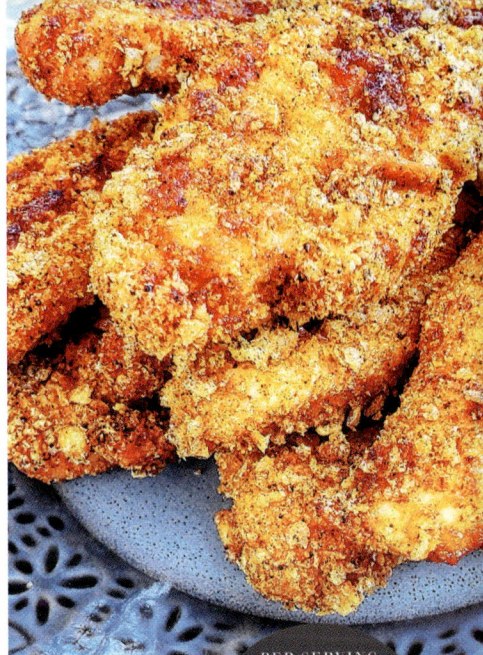

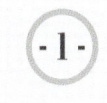
DIFFICULTY
-1-

SERVINGS
3

TIME
PREPARATION
25 MINS
COOKING
20 MINS

-PER SERVING-
538 CALORIES
PROTEIN: 70G
CARBS: 1G
FATS: 28G

INGREDIENTS

1 Lb of Chicken Tenderloins
1½ Cup of Pork Panko by Bacon's Heir
1 Tsp of Redmond Real Salt
1 Tsp of Paprika
¼ Tsp of Fresh Cracked Black Pepper

STEPS

- 1 - In a bowl, mix together the Pork Panko and seasonings.

- 2 - Place one chicken tenderloin at a time into the "breading" and pat the Pork Panko mixture into the chicken until fully coated on all sides.

- 3 - Set to the side while completing this process with all tenderloins.

- 4 - Heat air fryer to 390°F.

- 5 - Place the chicken tenders into the air fryer and cook for 20 minutes.

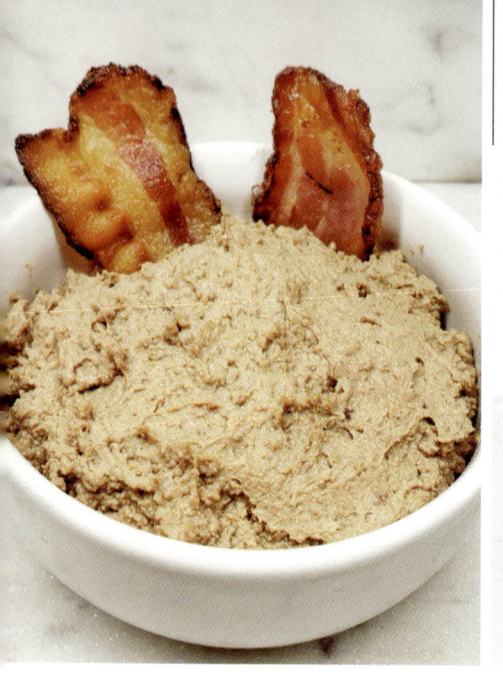

BACON FAT CHICKEN LIVER PÂTÉ

TIME — SERVINGS — DIFFICULTY

PREPARATION 20 MINS
COOKING 20 MINS

SERVINGS: 8

-PER SERVING-
179 CALORIES
PROTEIN: 10G
CARBS: 0G
FATS: 16G

INGREDIENTS

1 Lb of Chicken Livers
½ Cup of Bacon Fat
1 Tsp of Redmond Real Salt

STEPS

- 1 - Heat a cast iron skillet or nonstick pan to medium-high heat with ¼ cup of bacon fat.

- 2 - Add the chicken livers and sear on both sides for 3 to 5 minutes.

- 3 - Pour everything in the pan into a food processor and pulse.

- 4 - Slowly add the other ¼ cup of bacon fat to the food processor and continue to pulse until blended smooth.

STEAK TACOS

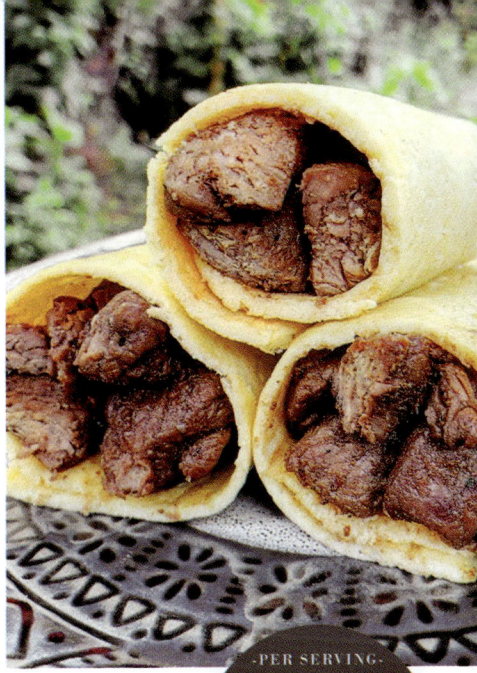

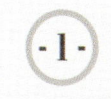  

DIFFICULTY -1-

SERVINGS 2

TIME
PREPARATION 10 MINS
COOKING 15 MINS

PER SERVING
504 CALORIES
PROTEIN: 46G
CARBS: 0G
FATS: 35G

INGREDIENTS

1 Lb Top Sirloin Steak
1 Tbsp of Fat of Choice
1 Tsp of Redmond Real Salt
½ Tsp of Ground Cumin
¼ Tsp of Crushed Red Pepper

STEPS

- 1 - Heat a cast-iron skillet or nonstick pan to medium high heat with fat of choice.

- 2 - Add steak to the pan.

- 3 - Quickly sear on both sides.

- 4 - Remove from the pan and cut into 2-inch pieces.

- 5 - Place the steak pieces back on the pan and add seasonings over top.

The Ultimate Carnivore Cookbook / 75
www.bioptimizedketo.com

STEAK TACOS

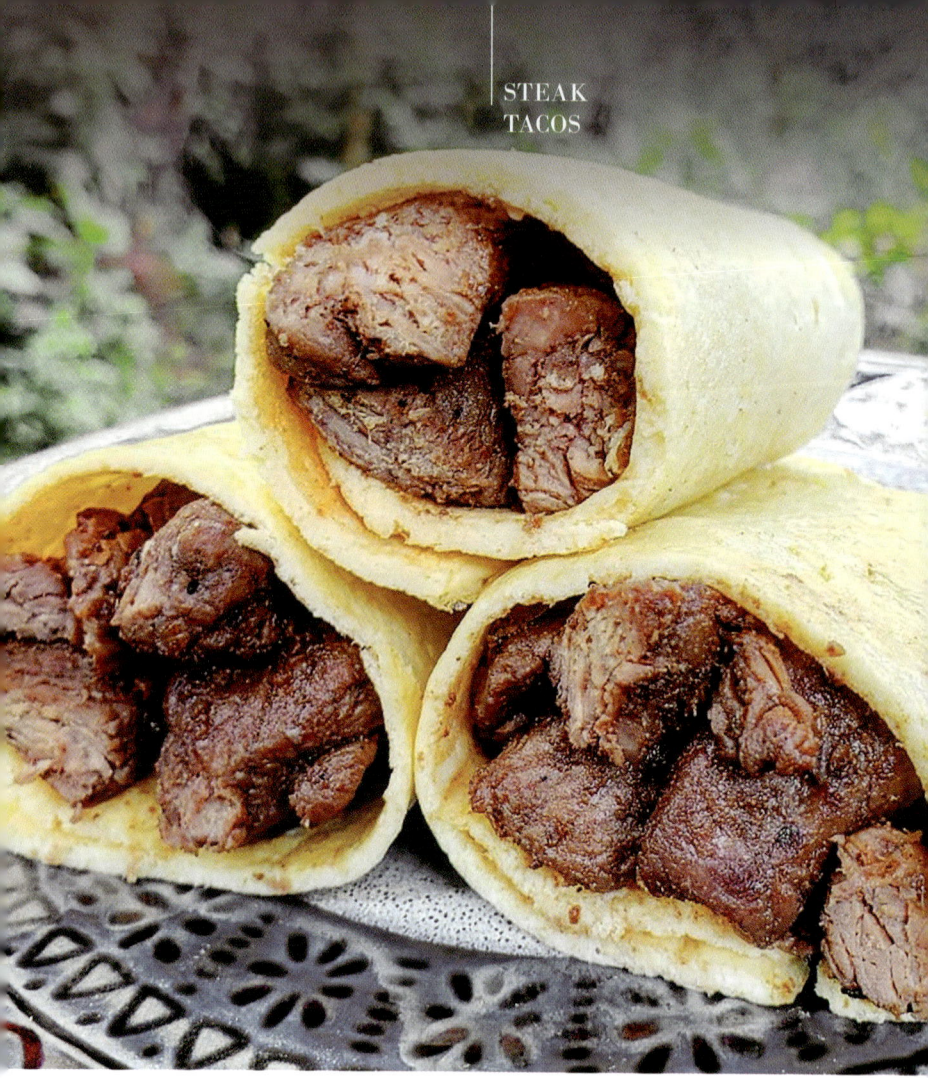

STEPS

- 6 - Work steak pieces around the pan cooking and adding the flavor of the seasonings.

- 7 - Once browned on all sides, remove and place inside of Carnivore Tortillas.* (See recipe)

OVEN ROASTED BABY BACK RIBS

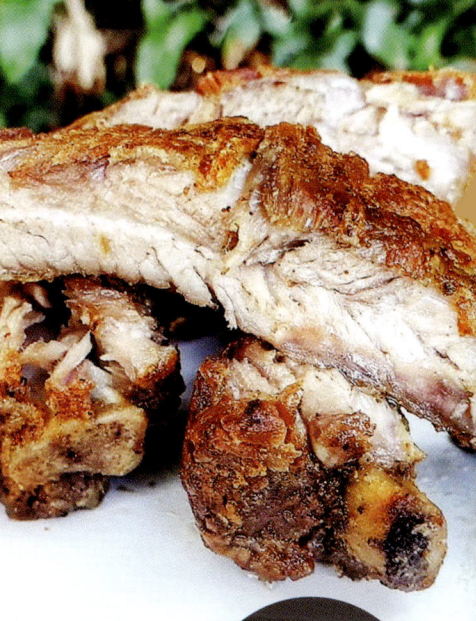

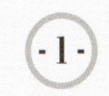
DIFFICULTY

SERVINGS
4

TIME
PREPARATION
2½ HOURS

COOKING
3 HOURS

PER SERVING
261 CALORIES
PROTEIN: 15G
CARBS: 1G
FATS: 22G

INGREDIENTS

1 Rack of Pork Ribs (approximately 2 Lbs)
1½ Tsp of Redmond Real Salt
1 Tsp of Fresh Cracked Black Pepper
1 Tsp of Ground Cinnamon (Optional)
1 Tsp of Allspice (Optional)

STEPS

- 1 - Start by pat drying the pork ribs and placing them on a wire rack above a baking pan.

- 2 - Apply a layer of salt to the top side of the ribs and the salt.

    Note Do not rub the salt in.

- 3 - Place in the refrigerator for at least 2 hours.

- 4 - Remove from the refrigerator and rinse the salt off.

The Ultimate Carnivore Cookbook /
www.bioptimizedketo.com

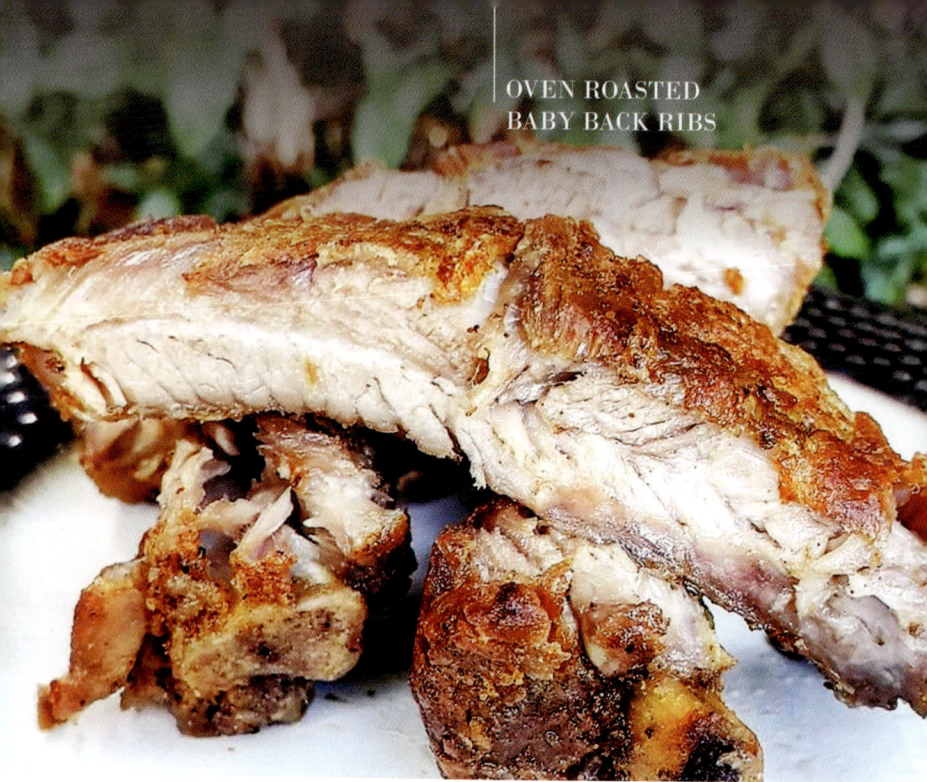

OVEN ROASTED BABY BACK RIBS

STEPS

- 5 - Preheat the oven to 275°F.
- 6 - Pat dry the water off and season on all sides with salt, pepper, cinnamon, and allspice.
- 7 - Wrap in aluminum foil and place back on to the wire rack.
- 8 - Put the ribs into the oven and set a timer for 2 hours.
- 9 - After the 2 hours, turn the heat up to 350°F.
- 10 - Once the oven reaches 350°F set the timer for 30 more minutes.
- 11 - Remove from the oven and let rest for 20 minutes before unwrapping.
- 12 - Cut between each bone and serve.

CHICKEN & CHEESE PIZZA CRUST

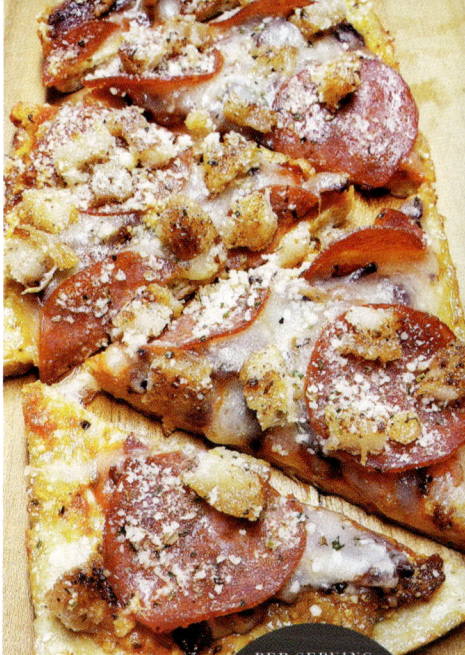

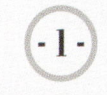

DIFFICULTY: 1
SERVINGS: 2
TIME:
PREPARATION 20 MINS
COOKING 20 MINS

·PER SERVING·
394 CALORIES
PROTEIN: 44G
CARBS: 1G
FATS: 24G

INGREDIENTS

1 Lb of Ground Chicken
3 Oz of Shredded Cheese
2 Tsp of Garlic & Herb Seasonings
1 Tsp of Redmond Real Salt

STEPS

- 1 -   Preheat the oven to 400°F.

- 2 -   Mix all ingredients thoroughly in a bowl.

- 3 -   Pack mixture thinly in a baking sheet lined with aluminum foil.

- 4 -   Place into the oven and bake for 15 minutes.

Note The crust will shrink a small amount.

CHICKEN & CHEESE PIZZA CRUST

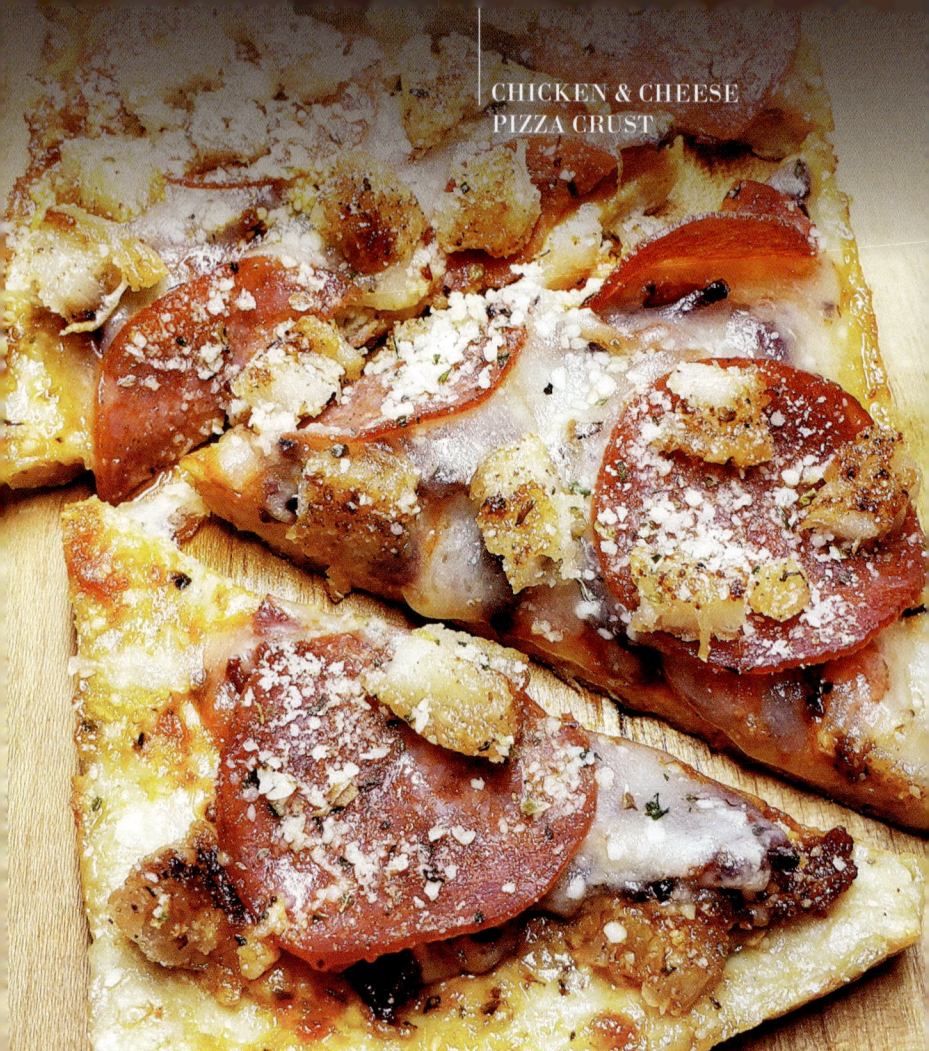

STEPS

- 5 -   Remove from the oven and top with desired toppings and cheeses.

- 6 -   Return to the oven for 5 more minutes.

- 7 -   Once cheese has melted, take out of the oven to be cut and served.

ROASTED BONE MARROW

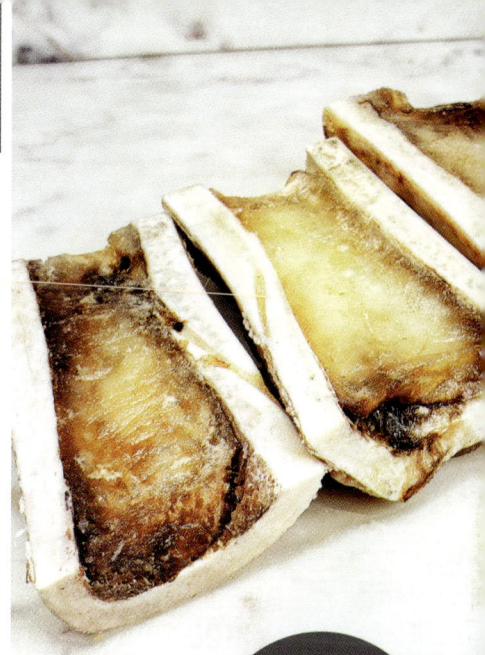

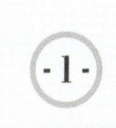  

DIFFICULTY: 1
SERVINGS: 2
TIME: PREPARATION 5 MINS / COOKING 25 MINS

-PER SERVING-
315 CALORIES
PROTEIN: 0G
CARBS: 0G
FATS: 35G

INGREDIENTS

Canoe Cut Marrow Bones (approximately 2½ Lbs)
½ Tsp of Redmond Real Salt

STEPS

- 1 - Preheat the oven to 400°F.

- 2 - Lay marrow bones on a baking sheet lined with aluminum foil.

- 3 - Sprinkle the tops with salt.

- 4 - Place into the oven and roast for 25 minutes or until the marrow starts to leak from the bones.

- 5 - Serve immediately after removing from the oven.

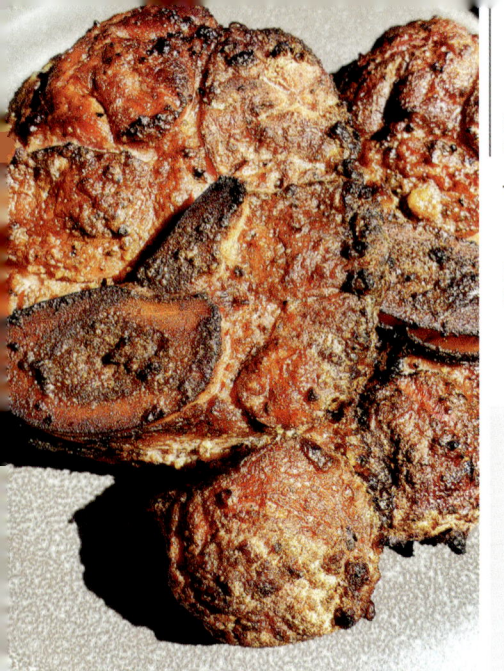

SMOKED VEAL SHANKS

TIME	SERVINGS	DIFFICULTY
PREPARATION 20 MINS COOKING 1-2 HOURS	2	

-PER SERVING-

243 CALORIES

PROTEIN: 44G
CARBS: 0G
FATS: 8G

INGREDIENTS

1 Lb of Veal Shanks
1 Tsp of Redmond Real Salt
½ Tsp of Fresh Cracked Black Pepper

STEPS

- 1 -   Heat smoker to 220°F.

- 2 -   Season veal shanks on both sides with salt and pepper.

- 3 -   Smoke until the internal temperature reaches 165°F.

- 4 -   Cut into pieces and serve with the bones.

PAN SEARED EGG YOLKS

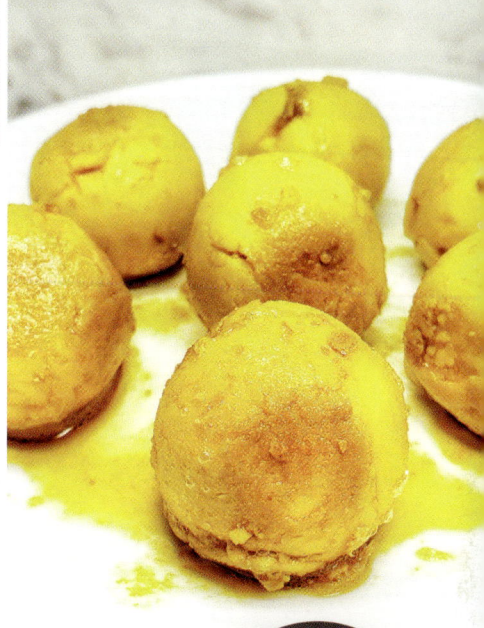

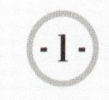  

DIFFICULTY: 1
SERVINGS: 3
TIME: PREPARATION 20 MINS / COOKING 15 MINS

-PER SERVING-
185 CALORIES
PROTEIN: 15G
CARBS: 1G
FATS: 14G

INGREDIENTS

7 Large Eggs
1 Tsp of Redmond Real Salt
1½ Tsp of Garlic Ghee* (see recipe)

STEPS

- 1 - Start by hard boiling the eggs.

- 2 - Once boiled, cool the eggs.

- 3 - Peel the eggs and carefully remove the yolks.

- 4 - Heat a nonstick pan to medium-low heat with the Garlic Ghee.

- 5 - Add the yolks to the pan and roll around being careful to not damage the yolks.

The Ultimate Carnivore Cookbook / 83
www.bioptimizedketo.com

PAN SEARED EGG YOLKS

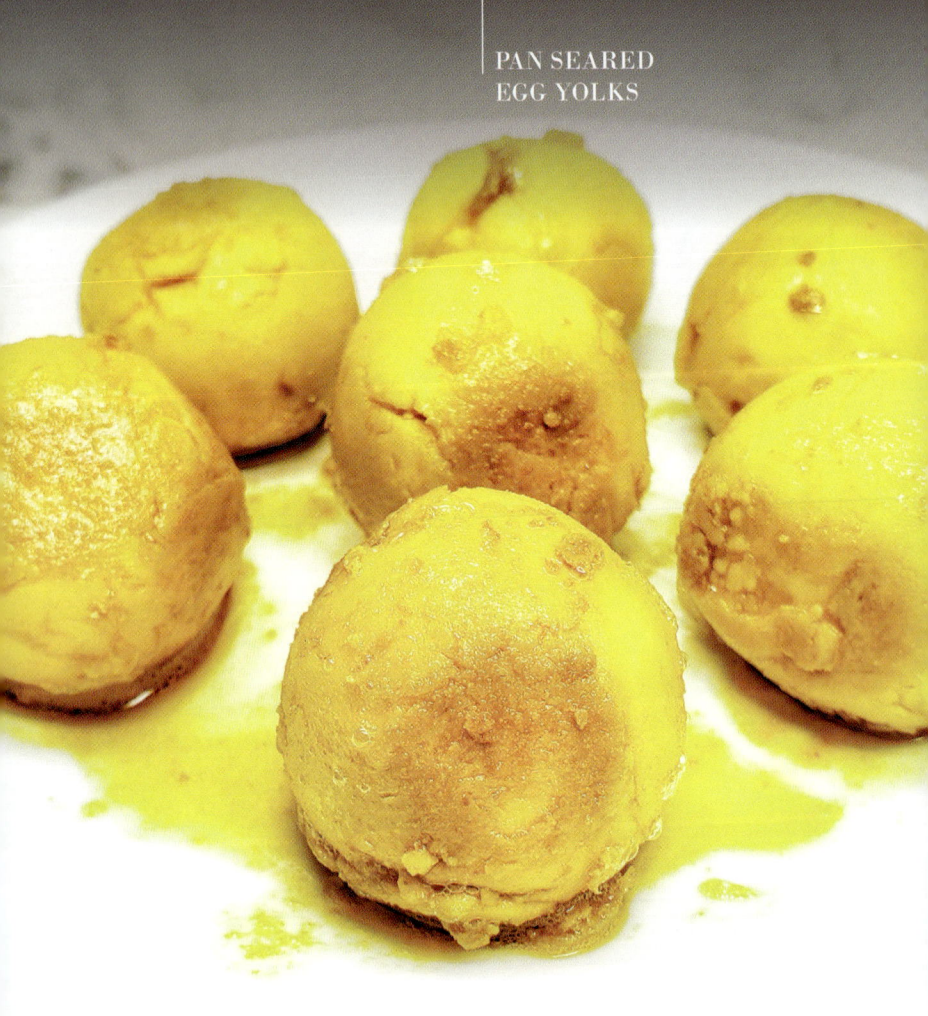

STEPS

- 6 - Cook until yolks start to brown.

- 7 - Remove from the pan and pour the remaining Garlic Ghee over the tops of the yolks.

HERB CRUSTED LAMB CHOPS

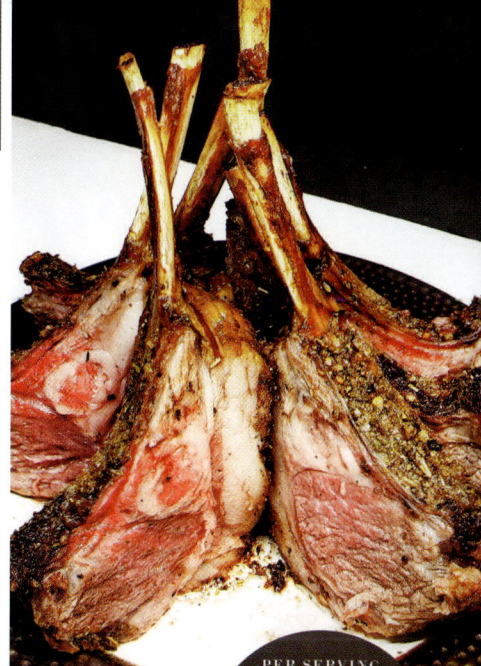

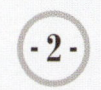 

DIFFICULTY: -2-

SERVINGS: 6

TIME: PREPARATION 30 MINS / COOKING 1½ HOURS

-PER SERVING-
492 CALORIES
PROTEIN: 21G
CARBS: 0G
FATS: 45G

INGREDIENTS

- 1 Rack of Lamb (approximately 1½ Lb)
- 1 Cup of Softened Butter or Ghee
- 2 Tsp of Redmond Real Salt
- 1 Tsp of Fresh Cracked Black Pepper
- ½ Tsp of Garlic Flakes
- ½ Tsp of Rosemary
- ½ Tsp of Thyme
- ½ Tsp of Oregano
- ½ Tsp of Onion Powder

STEPS

- 1 - Preheat oven to 500°F.
- 2 - Layer butter or ghee all over the lamb.
- 3 - Mix all seasonings together in a bowl.
- 4 - Sprinkle seasonings evenly on top of the butter/ghee layer.

HERB CRUSTED LAMB CHOPS

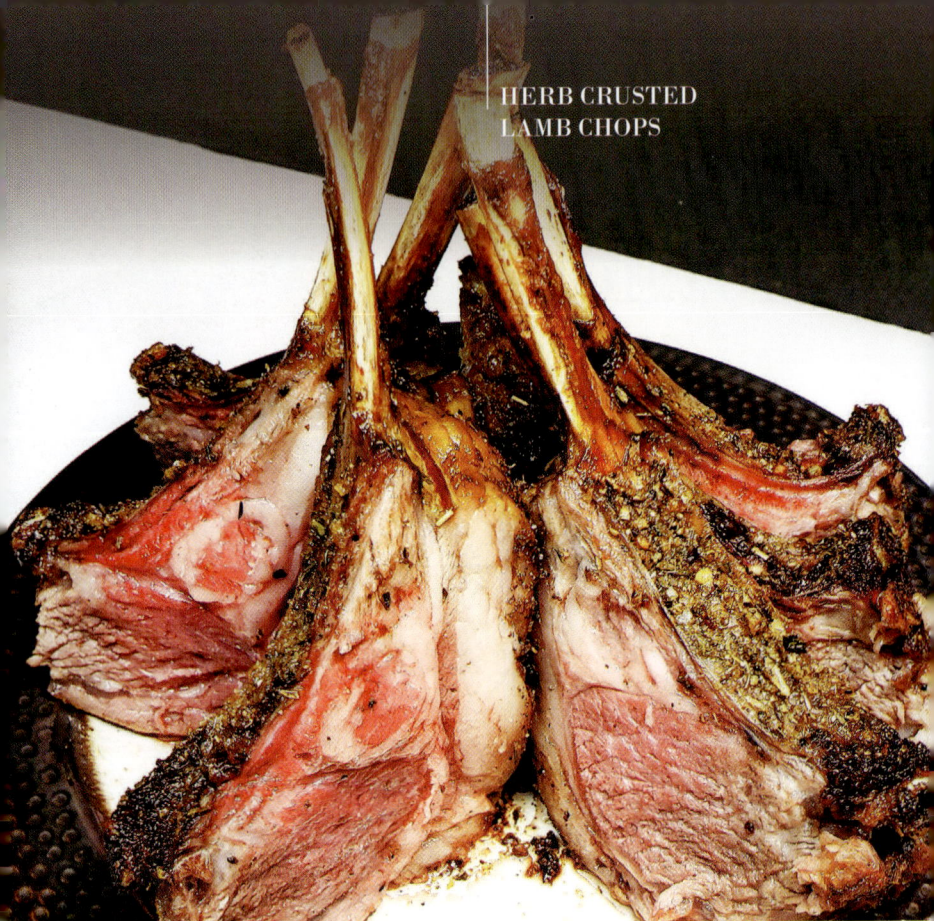

STEPS

- 5 - On a baking sheet lined with aluminum foil, place the rack of lamb.

- 6 - Put into the oven and cook for 15 minutes then turn the oven temperature down to 325°F.

- 7 - Continue cooking inside of the oven until the internal temperature reaches 145°F.

- 8 - Remove from the oven and then let rest for 10 minutes before slicing between the bones.

CRUNCHY CHEESE SHELL TACOS

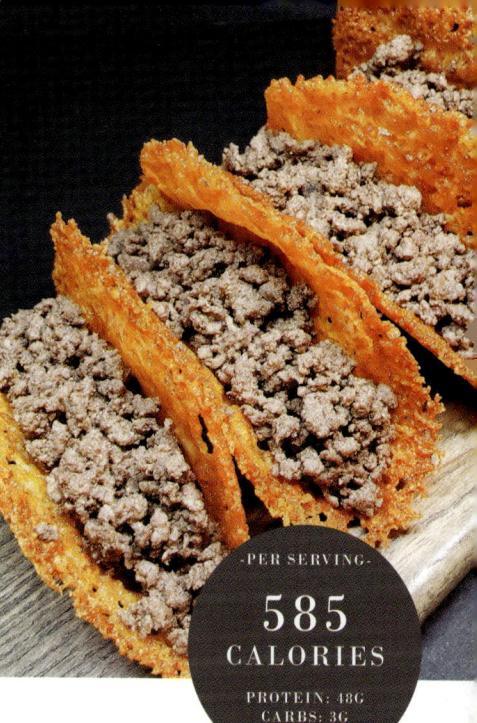

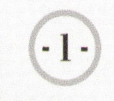
DIFFICULTY
-1-

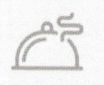
SERVINGS
4

TIME
PREPARATION 20 MINS
COOKING 35 MINS

-PER SERVING-
585 CALORIES
PROTEIN: 48G
CARBS: 3G
FATS: 42G

INGREDIENTS

- 2 Lbs of Ground Beef (85/15)
- 8 Oz of Shredded Cheese
- ¼ Cup of Water
- 1 Tbsp of Chili Powder
- 2 Tsp of Ground Cumin
- 1 Tsp of Redmond Real Salt
- 1 Tsp of Fresh Cracked Black Pepper
- ½ Tsp of Paprika
- ½ Tsp of Garlic Powder
- ¼ Tsp of Onion Powder

STEPS

- 1 - Heat a nonstick pan to a medium temperature.

- 2 - Place a long-handled kitchen utensil on the top of a bowl.

  Note This will be for shaping the cheese into a taco shell.

- 3 - Add shredded cheese to the pan and spread thinly with a spatula.

- 4 - Cook until the cheese becomes crispy almost completely.

The Ultimate Carnivore Cookbook / 87
www.bioptimizedketo.com

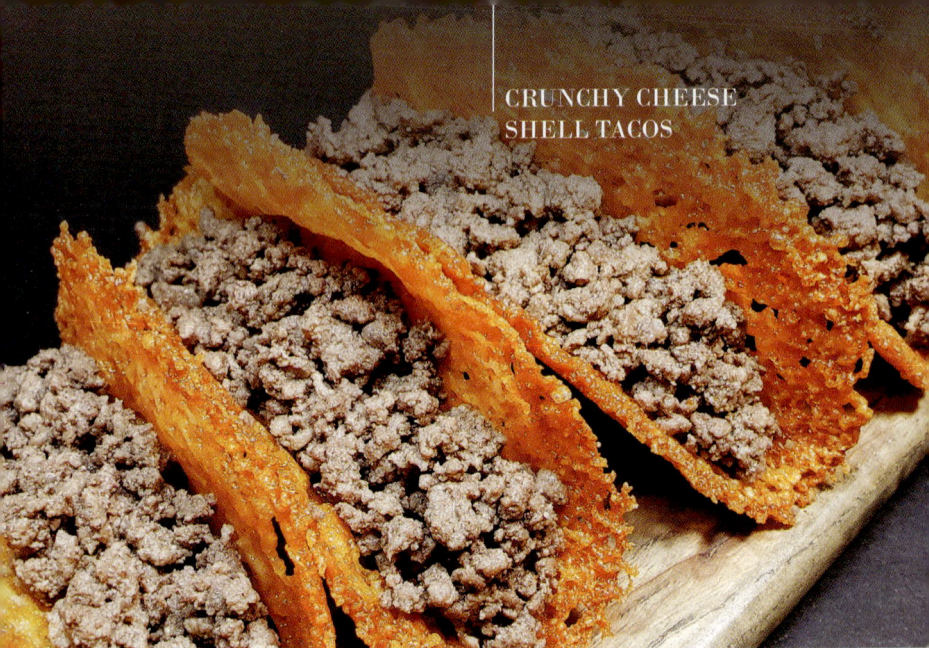

CRUNCHY CHEESE SHELL TACOS

STEPS

- 5 - Remove from the pan with the spatula and drape over top of the handle of the kitchen utensil that has been placed over a bowl.

- 6 - Repeat this process until all cheese has been turned into taco shells.

- 7 - In the same pan, add the ground beef and turn the heat up to a medium high temperature.

- 8 - Break the meat up with the spatula by stirring in the pan.

- 9 - Mix seasonings in a bowl and add them to the pan with the ground beef.

- 10 - Mix the seasonings into the meat and then add the water.

- 11 - Stir together frequently while letting the water reduce.

- 12 - Cook until water has evaporated.

- 13 - Place inside of the Cheese Shells and serve.

BEEF WELLINGTON

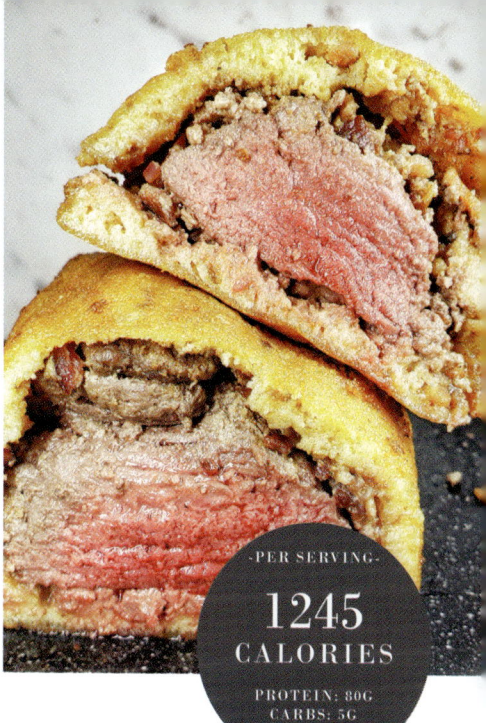

DIFFICULTY - 3 -

SERVINGS 4

TIME
PREPARATION 35 MINS
COOKING 25 MINS

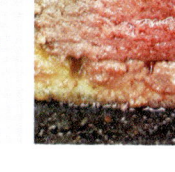
-PER SERVING-
1245 CALORIES
PROTEIN: 80G
CARBS: 5G
FATS: 101G

INGREDIENTS

1 Lb of Beef Tenderloin
1 Cup of Beef Or Chicken Liver Pâté*
  (see recipe)
1 Cup of Chopped Cooked Bacon
½ Tsp of Redmond Real Salt
½ Tsp of Fresh Cracked Black Pepper
4 Cups of Fat of Choice

PASTRY DOUGH INGREDIENTS
2 Cups of Pork Panko by
  Bacon's Heir
9 Tbsp of Egg Whites
2 Large Eggs

STEPS

- 1 -   Start by mixing the Pork Panko, eggs and egg whites in a large bowl.

- 2 -   In a separate bowl, mix together the Pâté and Chopped Bacon.

- 3 -   Heat a deep pot with fat of choice to medium-high heat.

- 4 -   Scoop the bacon and Pâté mixture on to the top of the beef tenderloin.

The Ultimate Carnivore Cookbook / 89
www.bioptimizedketo.com

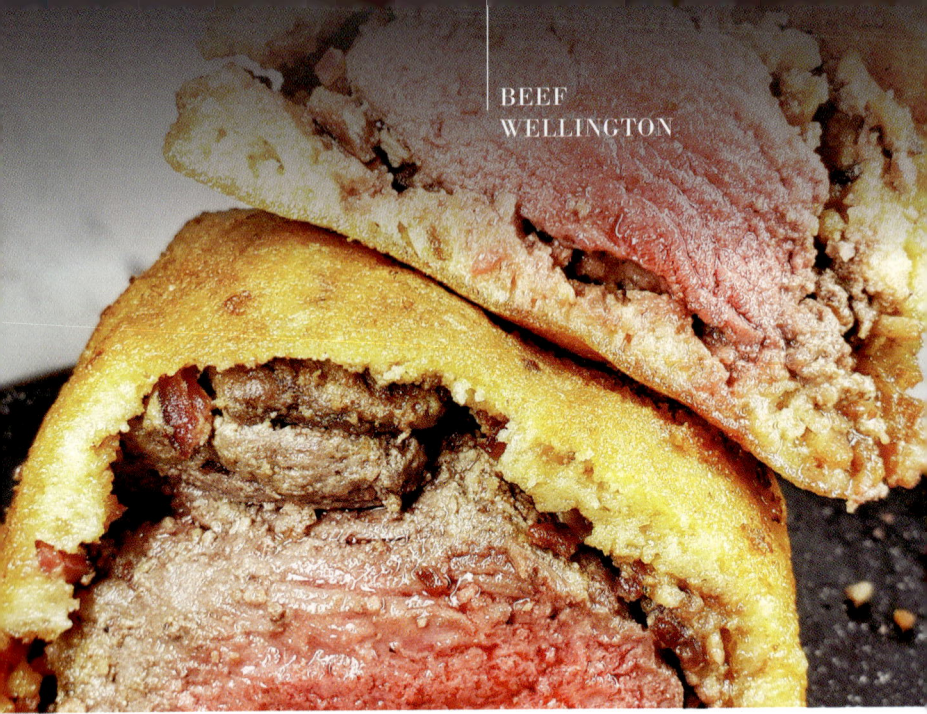

BEEF WELLINGTON

STEPS

- 5 - Place a layer of the Pastry Dough over the Pâté covered tenderloin.
- 6 - Roll on to the top side and repeat layering the Pâté and Pastry Dough over the bottom.
- 7 - Pack everything tightly around the tenderloin and seal the Pastry Dough on all sides.
- 8 - Place into the heated pot of fat.
- 9 - Roll the wellington over in the pot seconds after submerging to prevent the dough from cracking or separating.
- 10 - Cook for 15 minutes or until the dough has become golden brown and crispy all over.
- 11 - Remove from the pot and rest on a wire rack to drain excess fat and then serve.

BACON WRAPPED STRIP STEAK

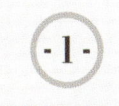
DIFFICULTY
· 1 ·

SERVINGS
4

TIME
PREPARATION
20 MINS
COOKING
25 MINS

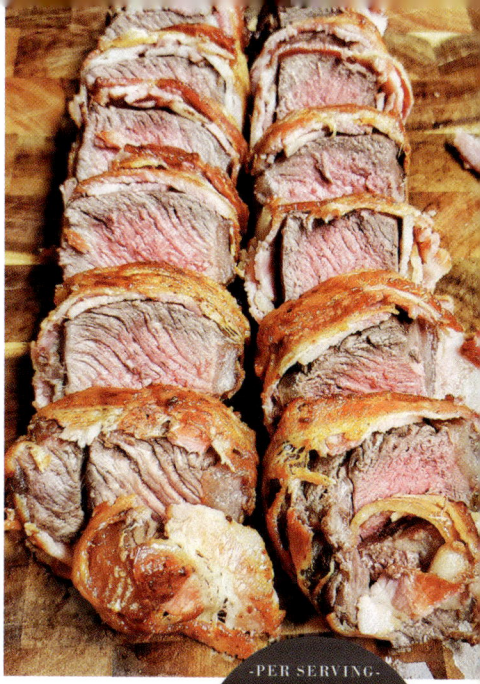

-PER SERVING-
568 CALORIES
PROTEIN: 33G
CARBS: 0G
FATS: 48G

INGREDIENTS

2 Strip Loin Steaks (approximately 10 Oz each)
2 8 Oz Packs of Sugar-Free Bacon
1½ Tsp of Redmond Real Salt
½ Tbsp of Fat of Choice

STEPS

- 1 - Season the tops and bottoms of the strip loins with the salt.
- 2 - Wrap each steak tightly with the bacon.
- 3 - Heat a cast-iron skillet or nonstick pan with fat of choice to medium-high heat.
- 4 - Place the wrapped steaks into the pan and cook until the bacon has become crispy.
- 5 - Flip the steaks over and repeat.

The Ultimate Carnivore Cookbook / 91
www.bioptimizedketo.com

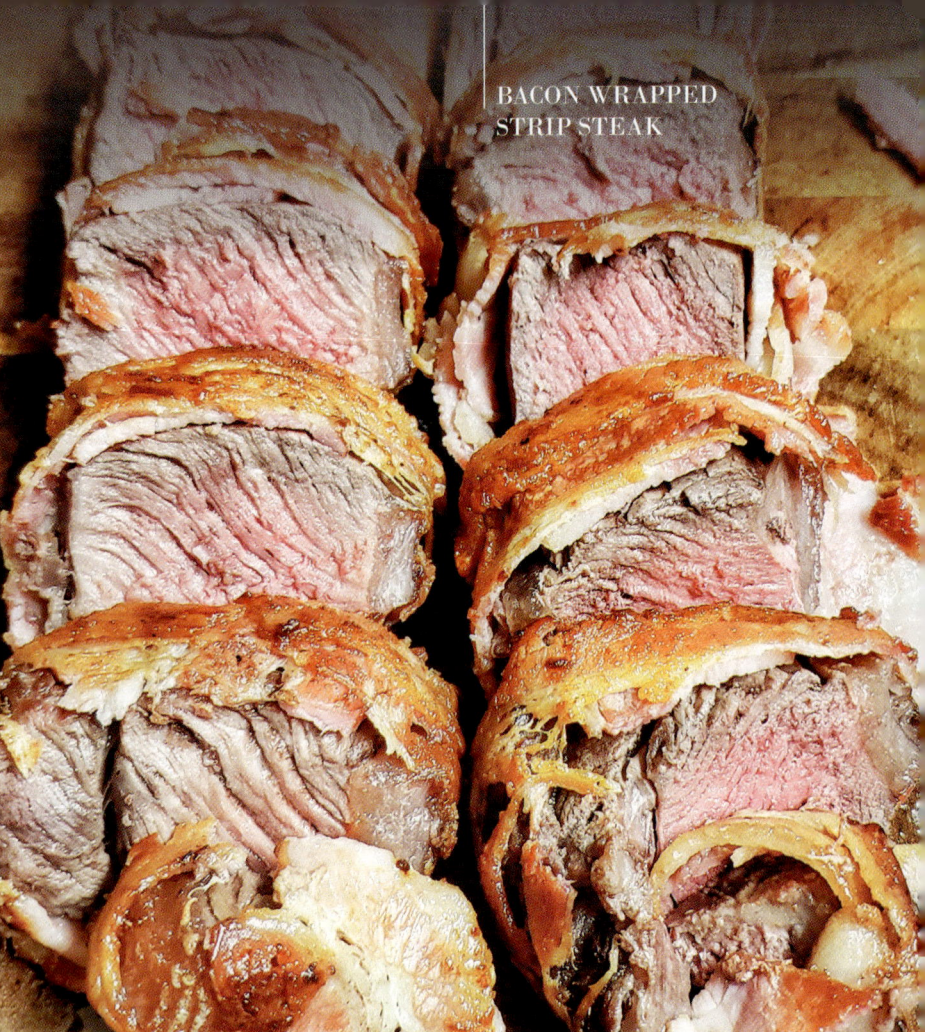

BACON WRAPPED STRIP STEAK

STEPS

- 6 - Once the tops and bottoms have become crispy, turn the steaks on to its side to cook.

- 7 - Do this to both sides and then remove from the pan.

- 8 - Cut and serve immediately after.

PRIMAL BLEND BURGER

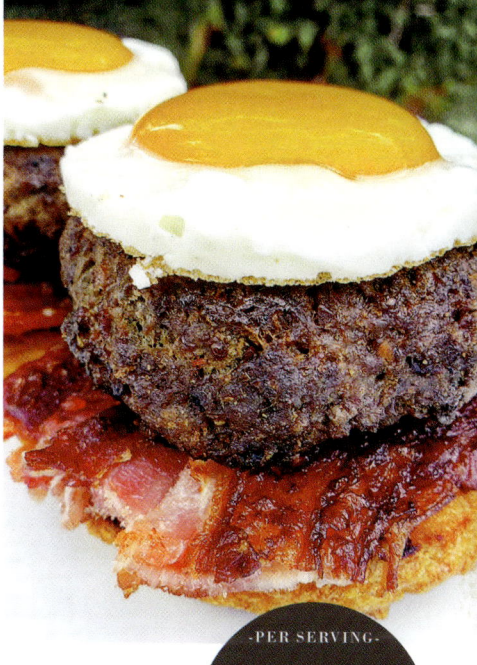

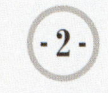
DIFFICULTY

SERVINGS
8

TIME
PREPARATION
35 MINS

COOKING
45 MINS

-PER SERVING-
391 CALORIES
PROTEIN: 44G
CARBS: 1G
FATS: 23G

INGREDIENTS

2 Lbs of Ground Beef (85/15)
1 Lb of Beef Heart
½ Lb of Beef Kidney
½ Lb of Beef Liver
1½ Tsp of Redmond Real Salt
1 Tsp of Fresh Cracked Black Pepper
1 Tbsp of Fat of Choice

STEPS

- 1 -   Cut beef kidney into cubes and the beef liver into strips.

- 2 -   Place the kidney and liver into a food processor or blender.

- 3 -   Pulse until it's chunky.

- 4 -   Cut beef heart into cubes and add those into the food processor/blender.

The Ultimate Carnivore Cookbook / 93
www.bioptimizedketo.com

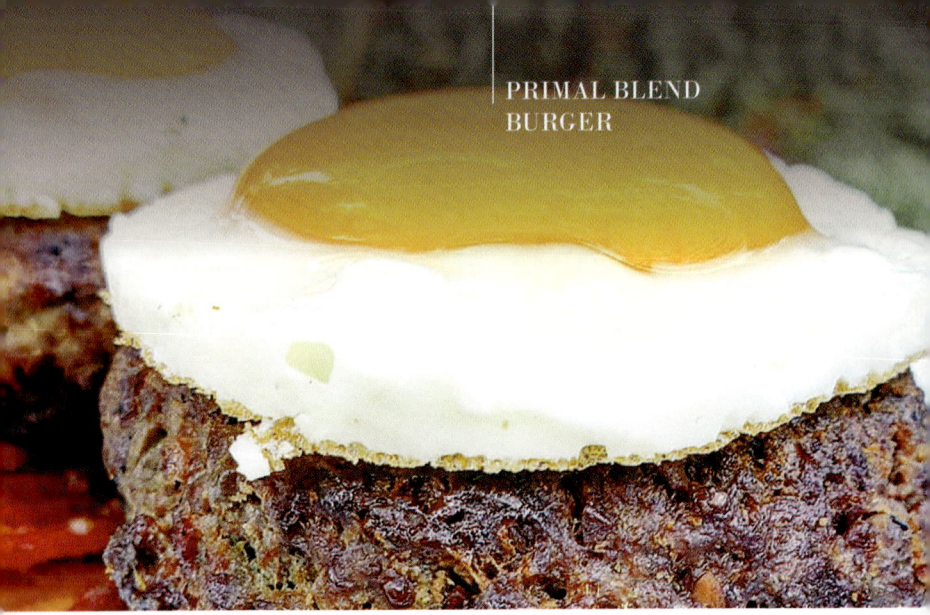

PRIMAL BLEND BURGER

STEPS

- 5 - Grind until mixture is similar to ground meat.

- 6 - In a large bowl, place the ground beef and add in the heart, kidney, and liver blend.

- 7 - Mix together thoroughly.

    Note Gloved hands work best to mix.

- 8 - After mixed, form into burger patties and set to the side on a piece of parchment paper.

- 9 - Season both sides of each burger patty with salt and pepper.

- 10 - Heat a cast iron skillet or nonstick pan with fat of choice to a medium-high heat.

- 11 - Place burger patties into the pan 2 to 3 at a time.

- 12 - Cook until the tops and bottoms have a hard sear.

- 13 - Place on Carnivore Buns* and top with desired toppings.

SLICED BEEF TONGUE

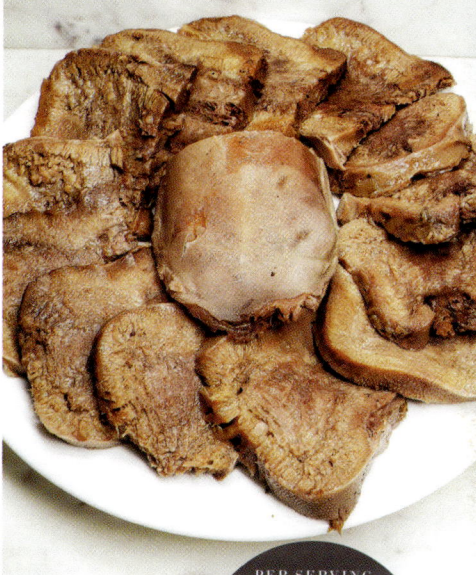

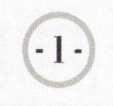
DIFFICULTY
- 1 -

SERVINGS
6

TIME
PREPARATION
20 MINS

COOKING
4-5 HOURS

-PER SERVING-
524 CALORIES
PROTEIN: 40G
CARBS: 8G
FATS: 37G

INGREDIENTS

1 Whole Beef Tongue (approximately 3 Lbs)
1½ Tsp of Redmond Real Salt
4 Cups of Bone Broth* (see recipe)

STEPS

- 1 -   Preheat the oven to 375°F.

- 2 -   Pour Bone Broth into a deep roasting pan.

- 3 -   Season the underside of the beef tongue with the salt.

- 4 -   Rest tongue into the roasting pan with the Bone Broth and cover with aluminum foil.

- 5 -   Roast in the covered pan for 4 to 5 hours.

The Ultimate Carnivore Cookbook
www.bioptimizedketo.com

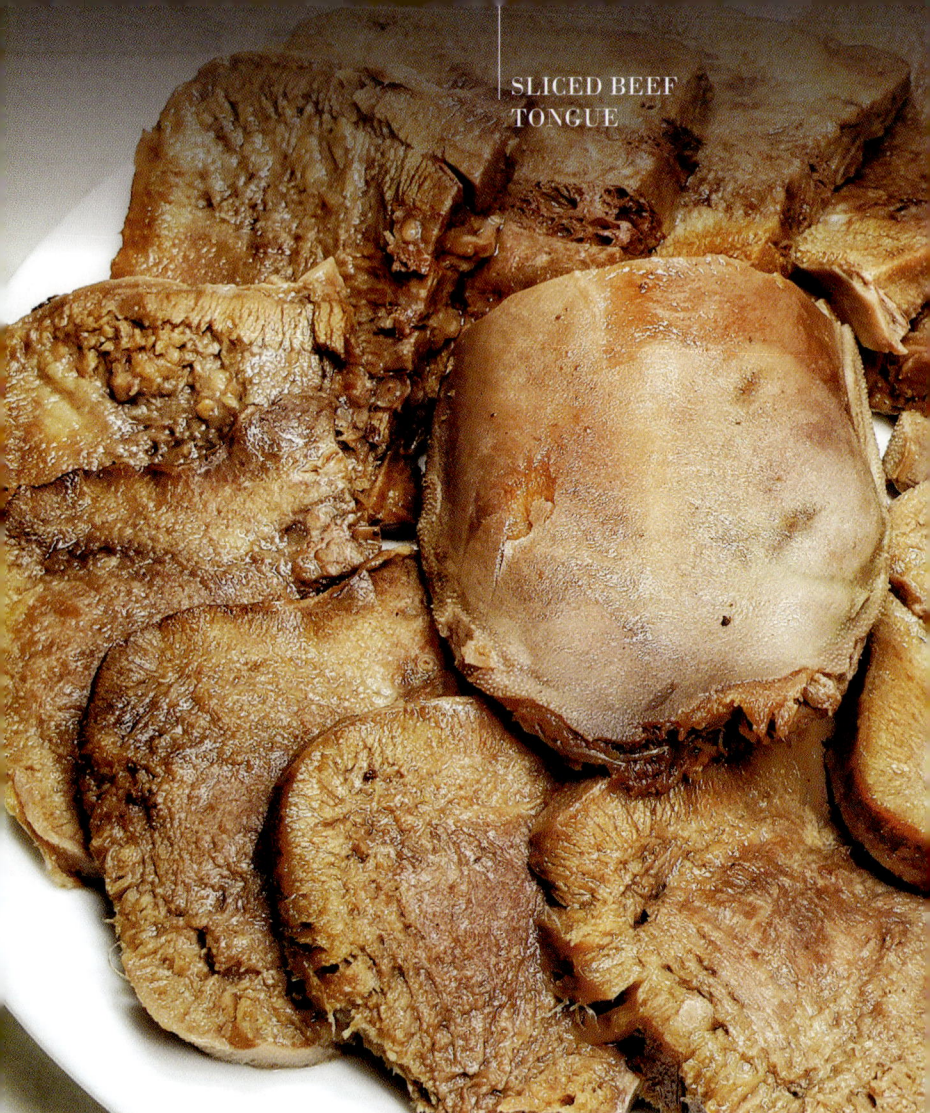

SLICED BEEF TONGUE

STEPS

- 6 - Remove from the oven and take out of the pan to cool enough to remove the skin.

- 7 - Slice across the tongue and serve.

BACON WRAPPED KIDNEY MEATBALLS

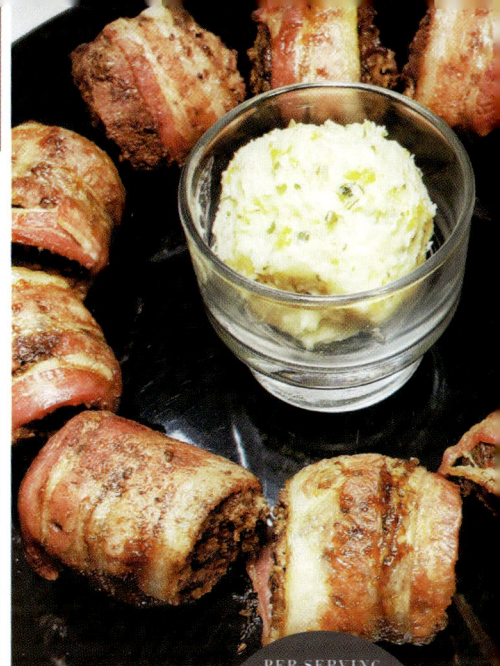

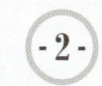

DIFFICULTY **SERVINGS** **TIME**
6
PREPARATION
40 MINS
COOKING
25 MINS

-PER SERVING-

538 CALORIES

PROTEIN: 46G
CARBS: 0G
FATS: 39G

INGREDIENTS

2 Lbs of Ground Beef (85/15)
1 8 Oz Pack of Sugar-Free Bacon
1 Lb of Beef Kidney
1½ Tsp of Redmond Real Salt
½ Tsp of Fresh Cracked Black Pepper

STEPS

- 1 - Cut the beef kidney into cubes and then place into a food processor or blender.

- 2 - Blend until nearly smooth.

- 3 - Add the ground beef into a large bowl and pour the blended kidney in.

- 4 - With gloved hands, mix together thoroughly.

- 5 - Lay the meat mixture flat on a piece of parchment paper.

The Ultimate Carnivore Cookbook / 97
www.bioptimizedketo.com

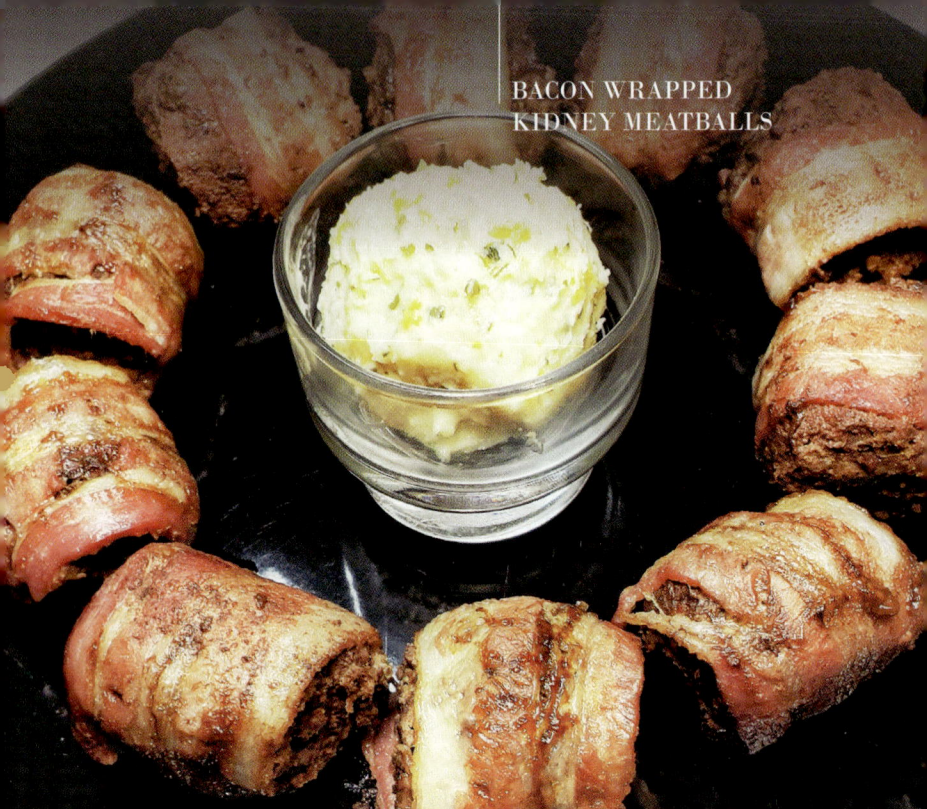

BACON WRAPPED KIDNEY MEATBALLS

STEPS

- 6 - Season evenly with salt and pepper.

- 7 - Roll into desired sizes and set to the side.

- 8 - Preheat the oven to 375°F.

- 9 - Cut bacon strips into 2 pieces.

- 10 - Wrap meatballs with the bacon pieces.

- 11 - Place meatballs on a baking sheet lined with aluminum foil and cook inside of the oven for 20 minutes.

- 12 - After the 20 minutes, place the meatballs under the broiler with it turned on for 5 minutes to crisp the bacon.

SALMON DIP

DIFFICULTY

SERVINGS
4

TIME
PREPARATION
25 MINS

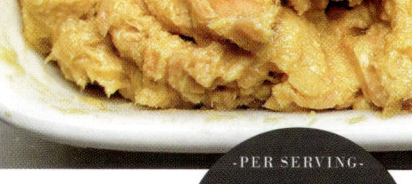

-PER SERVING-

323 CALORIES

PROTEIN: 43G
CARBS: 1G
FATS: 16G

INGREDIENTS

24 Oz of Cooked Salmon
½ Cup of Carnivore Mayo* (see recipe)
4 Yolks from Boiled Eggs

STEPS

- 1 -   In a large bowl, add the salmon and egg yolks.

- 2 -   Mix together by crushing the egg yolks into the salmon.

- 3 -   Add the mayo in and continue mixing thoroughly until everything is fully incorporated.

Note Add more mayo if necessary.

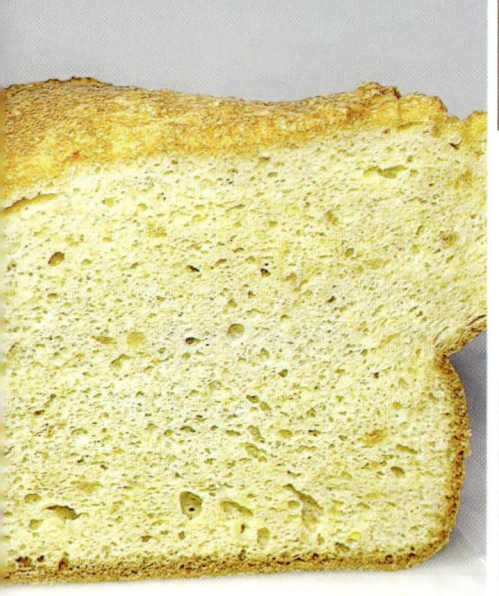

CARNIVORE BREAD

TIME
PREPARATION
30 MINS
COOKING
55 MINS

SERVINGS
10

DIFFICULTY
-1-

-PER SERVING-
383 CALORIES
PROTEIN: 36G
CARBS: 0G
FATS: 26G

INGREDIENTS

10 Large Eggs
70 Grams of Egg Whites
4 Cups of Pork Panko by Bacon's Heir
1-2 Tsp of Redmond Real Salt

STEPS

- 1 -   Start by separating the egg yolks from the egg whites into separate bowls.

        Note The bowl for the egg whites should be deep and large enough to whip the egg whites.

- 2 -   Add the additional egg whites to the bowl of separated egg whites.

- 3 -   Whip the egg whites until stiff peaks are formed then whip the egg yolks until smooth.

100 / The Ultimate Carnivore Cookbook
www.bioptimizedketo.com

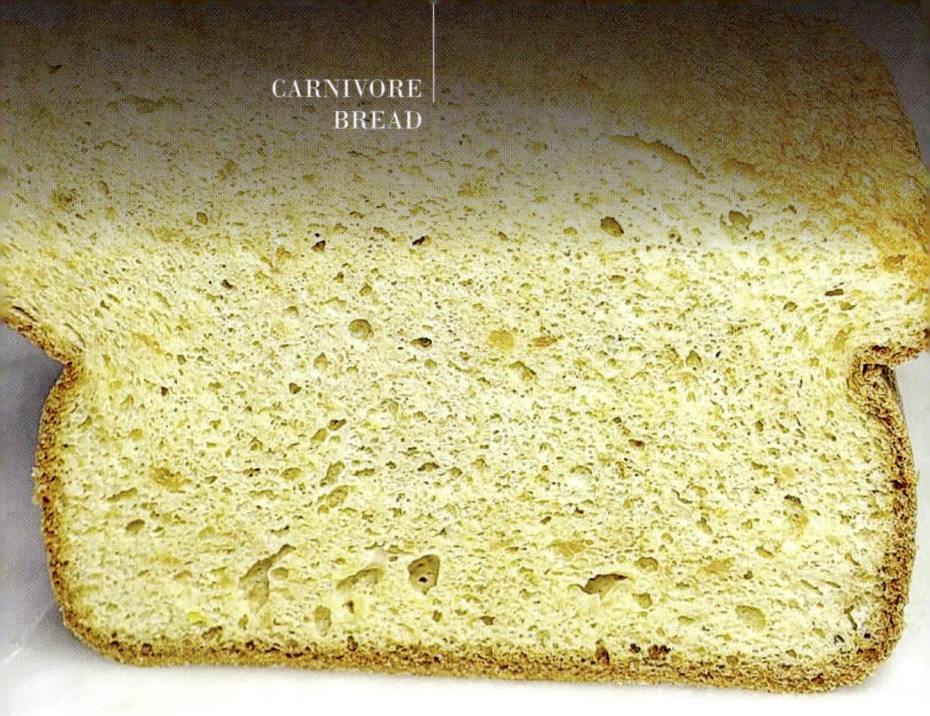

CARNIVORE BREAD

STEPS

- 4 - Add salt and Pork Panko into the bowl of egg whites.

- 5 - Mix together thoroughly.

    Note The egg whites will deflate as the Pork Panko gets mixed in.

- 6 - Pour the yolks into the mixture and stir into the batter until fully incorporated.

- 7 - Preheat the oven to 350°F.

- 8 - Place the batter into a 9"x5" size loaf pan and put the pan into the oven to bake for 55 minutes.

- 9 - Remove from the oven and let rest for 10 minutes before slicing.

    Note Can be refrigerated in an airtight container for 5 days or frozen for 3 months.

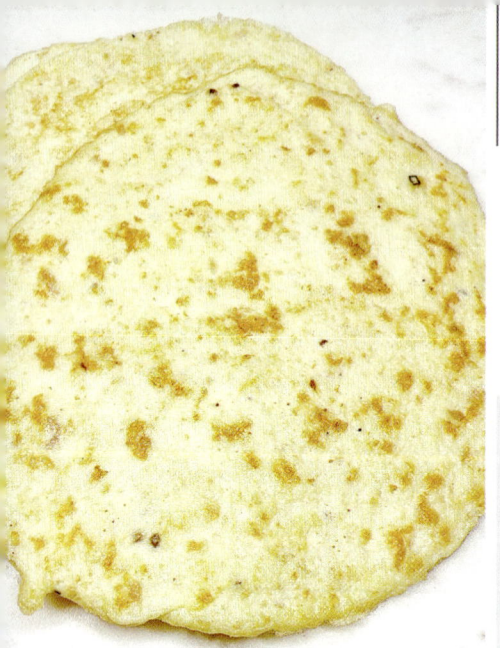

CARNIVORE TORTILLAS

TIME
PREPARATION 15 MINS
COOKING 30 MINS

SERVINGS 4

DIFFICULTY -1-

-PER SERVING-
170 CALORIES
PROTEIN: 11G
CARBS: 2G
FATS: 13G

INGREDIENTS

70 grams of Cooked White Meat Chicken
120 grams of Egg Whites
3 Tbsp of Pork Panko by Bacon's Heir
1 Tsp of Redmond Real Salt
1 Whole Large Egg

STEPS

- 1 -   Place all ingredients into a food processor or blender and blend until it's a smooth batter.

- 2 -   Heat a nonstick pan to medium low heat.

- 3 -   Pour a batter into the pan slowly and spread thinly with a spatula.

  Note The thinner the batter is spread, the better the end product will be.

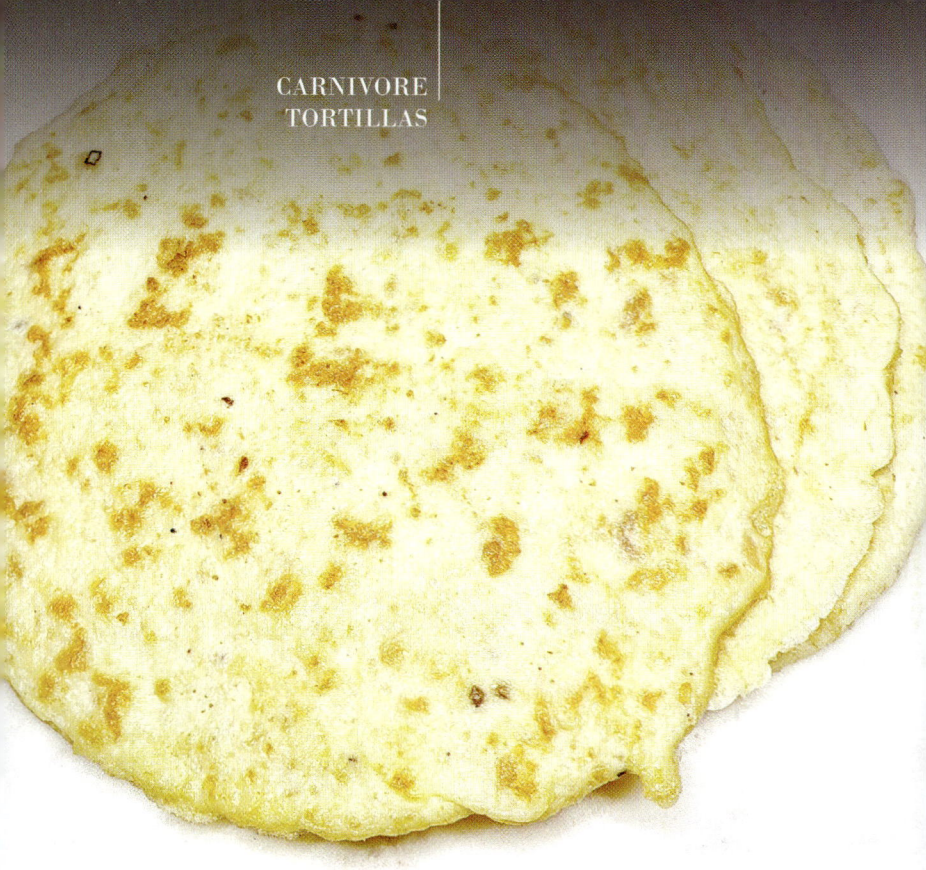

CARNIVORE TORTILLAS

STEPS

- 4 - Cook for 2 minutes or until the top side begins to cook, then flip over and cook for another 2 minutes.

    Note Each side should develop brown spots similar to a corn tortilla.

- 5 - Remove from the pan and place on the side until needed.

    Note Tortillas can be safely refrigerated for up to 5 days in an airtight container or frozen for 5 months.

    Note To reheat, place in a nonstick pan heated to medium low heat and cook until warm.

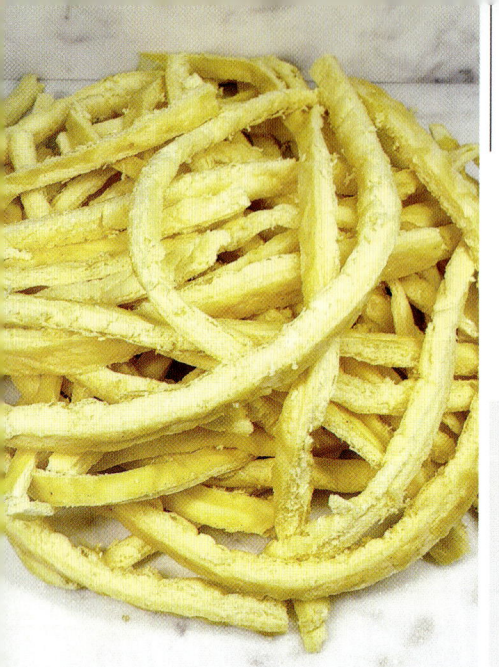

CARNIVORE NOODLES (DAIRY-FREE)

TIME   **SERVINGS**   **DIFFICULTY**

PREPARATION
15 MINS

COOKING
10 MINS

2

-PER SERVING-

234 CALORIES

PROTEIN: 37G
CARBS: 4G
FATS: 8G

INGREDIENTS

3 Large Eggs
3 Tbsp of Egg Whites
5 Tbsp of Whey Protein Isolate or Collagen Peptides
½ Tsp of Salt

STEPS

- 1 - Add all ingredients into a food processor or blender.

- 2 - Blend until the mixture is smooth.

- 3 - Preheat the oven to 350°F.

- 4 - Spread the batter thinly onto a baking sheet lined with parchment paper.

- 5 - Bake in the oven for 5 to 7 minutes.

CARNIVORE NOODLES
(DAIRY-FREE)

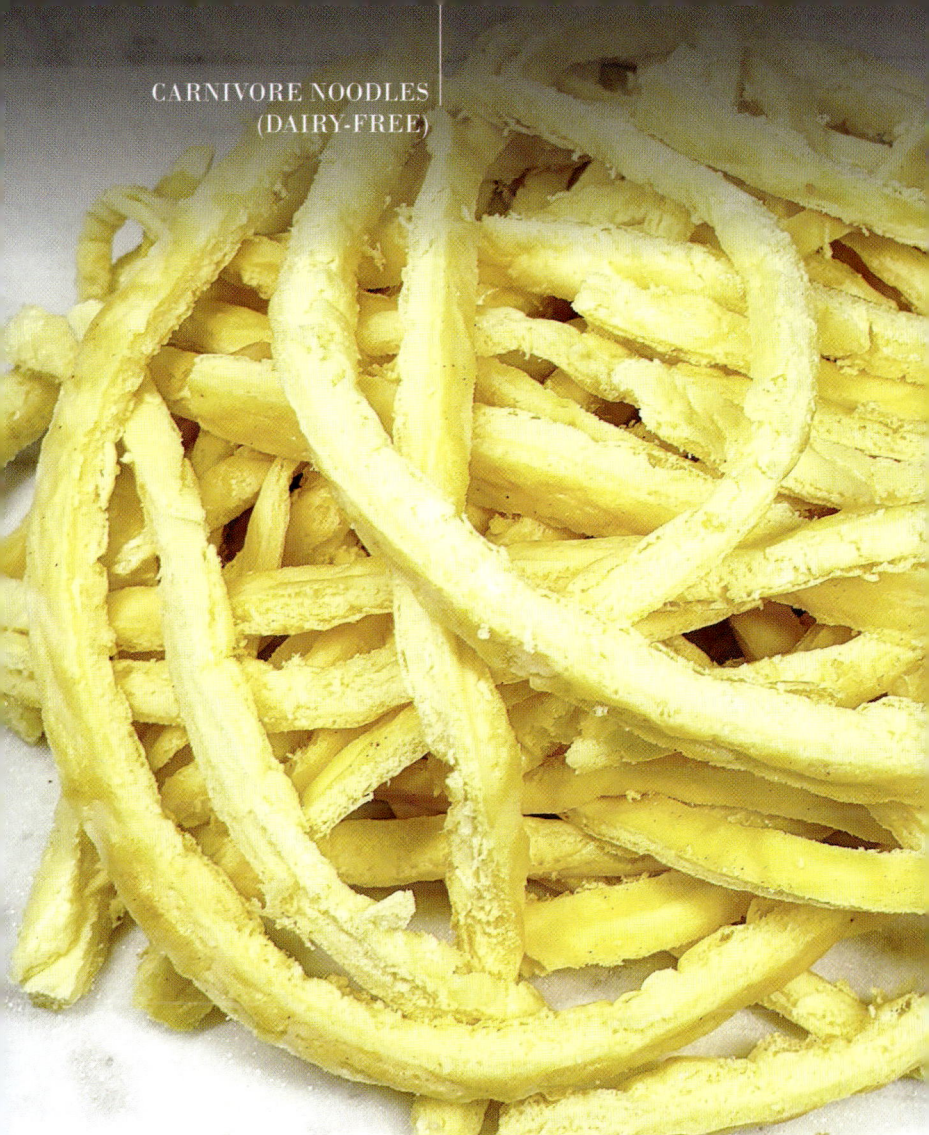

STEPS

- 6 - Pull out of the oven and let cool.

- 7 - Once cooled, cut into the length and width of the desired noodle size.

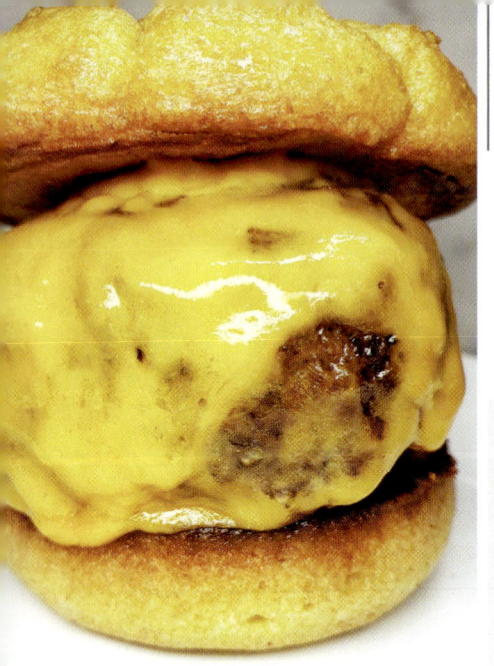

CARNIVORE BURGER BUN

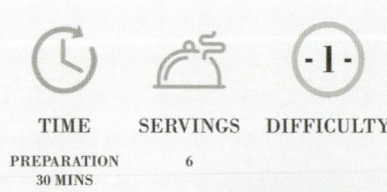

TIME
PREPARATION
30 MINS
COOKING
30 MINS

SERVINGS
6

DIFFICULTY
-1-

-PER SERVING-
319 CALORIES
PROTEIN: 30G
CARBS: 0G
FATS: 22G

INGREDIENTS

5 Large Eggs
30 Grams of Egg Whites
2 Cups of Pork Panko by Bacon's Heir
1 Tsp of Redmond Real Salt

STEPS

- 1 - Start by separating the egg yolks from the egg whites into separate bowls.

- 2 - The bowl for the egg whites should be large.

- 3 - Add the 30 grams of egg whites to the egg white bowl.

- 4 - Whip the egg whites into stiff peaks and whip the egg yolks until smooth.

- 5 - Add salt and Pork Panko into the bowl of egg whites and mix together thoroughly.

CARNIVORE BURGER BUN

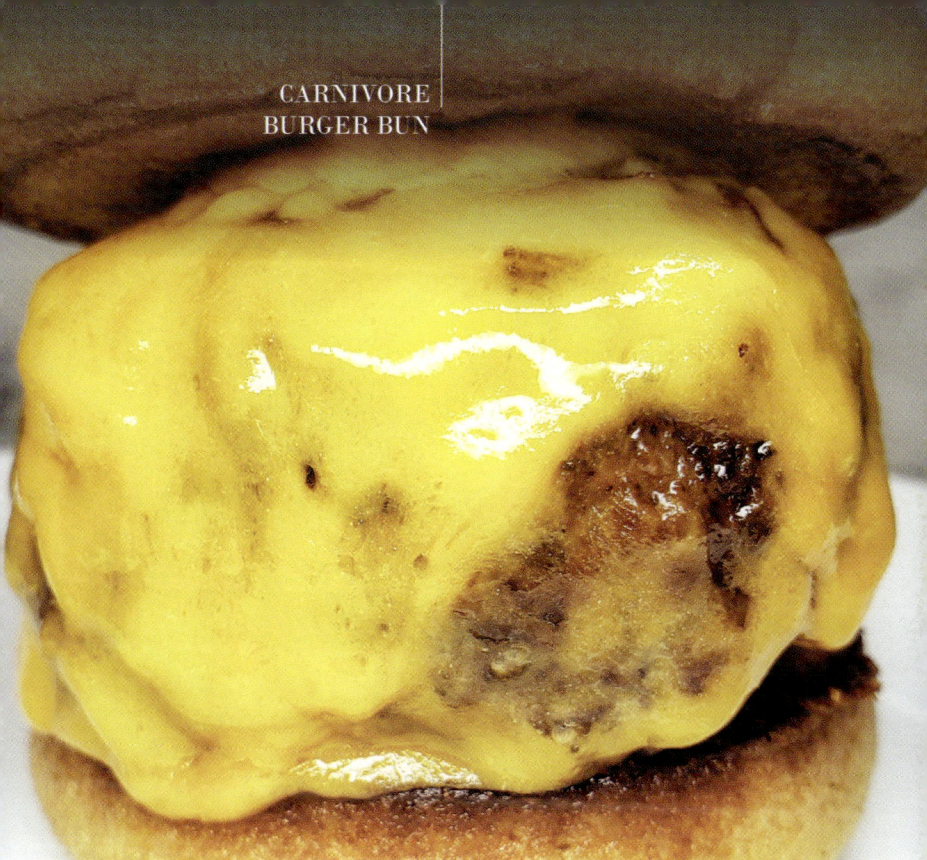

STEPS

- 6 - Pour the egg yolks into the mixture and stir into the batter until fully incorporated.

- 7 - Preheat the oven to 350°F.

- 8 - Add the batter into mini cake pans or a bun/biscuit pan.

- 9 - Bake for 30 minutes and take out of the oven.

- 10 - After removing from the oven, let rest inside the baking pan for 10 minutes before using it.

  Note Can be refrigerated in an airtight container for 5 days or frozen up to 3 months.

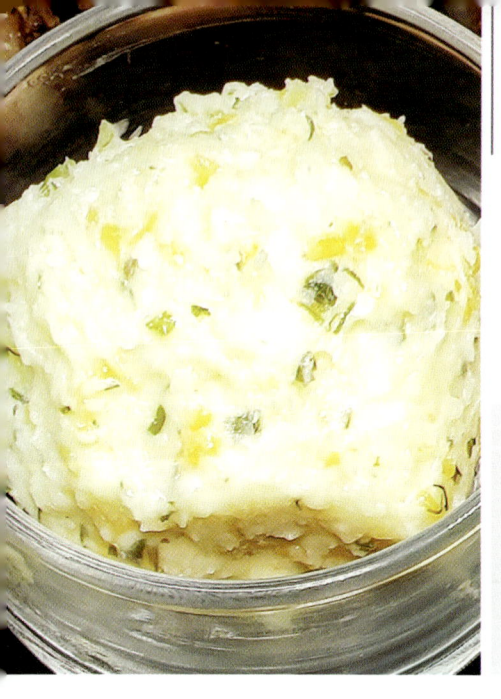

3 CHEESE BUTTER

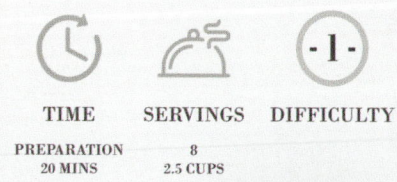

TIME
PREPARATION
20 MINS

SERVINGS
8
2.5 CUPS

DIFFICULTY

-PER SERVING-

291 CALORIES

PROTEIN: 6G
CARBS: 0G
FATS: 30G

INGREDIENTS

1 Cup of Unsalted Butter
2 Oz of Manchego Cheese
2 Oz of Smoked Cheddar
2 Oz of Monterey Jack
1 Tsp of Redmond Real Salt
½ Tsp of Garlic Flakes
¼ Tsp of Chopped Chives
¼ Tsp of Parsley
⅛ Tsp Black Pepper

STEPS

- 1 -   Set butter out to softened.

- 2 -   Shred the cheese and mix together.

- 3 -   Place the softened butter in a bowl and add the cheese.

- 4 -   Mix together thoroughly and then add the seasonings.

108 / The Ultimate Carnivore Cookbook
www.bioptimizedketo.com

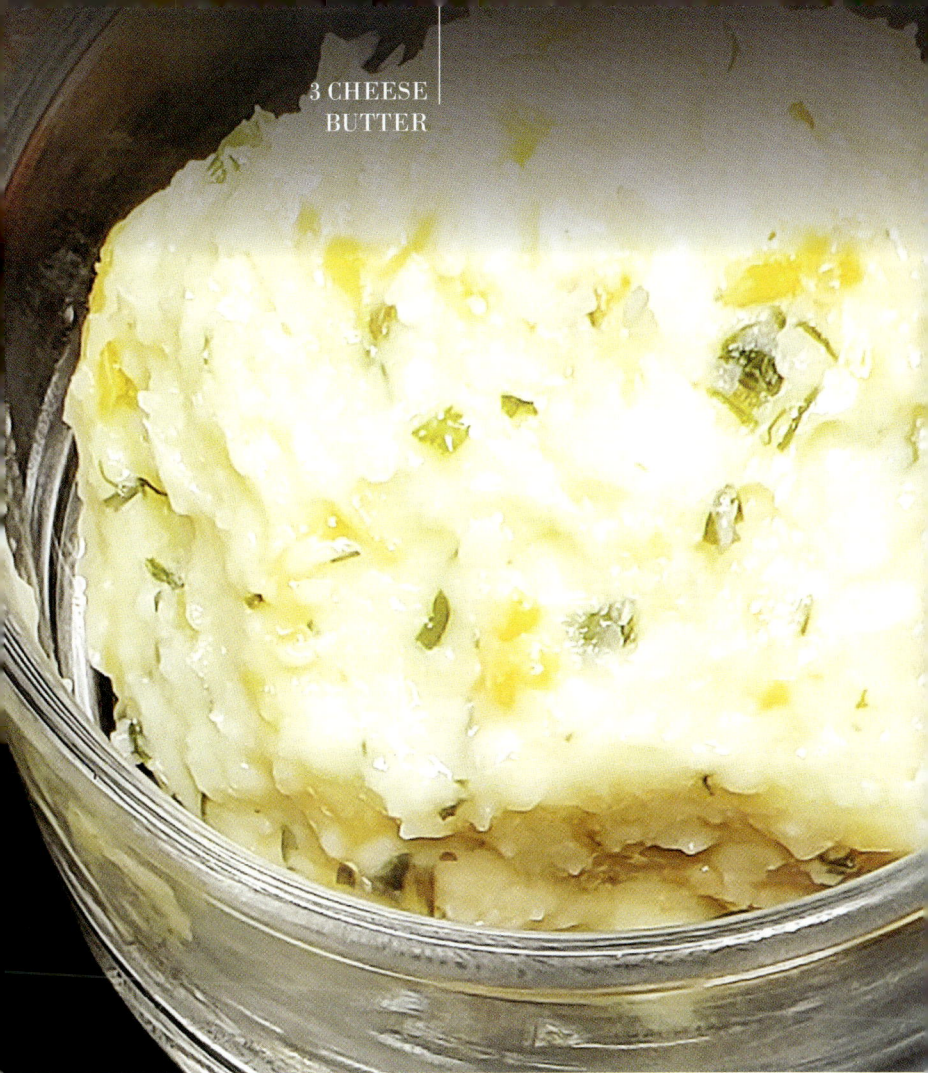

3 CHEESE BUTTER

STEPS

- 5 -   Mix again until everything is evenly incorporated.

- 6 -   Ready to use immediately.

Note Can be refrigerated in an airtight container for up to 7 days of can be frozen for 6 months.

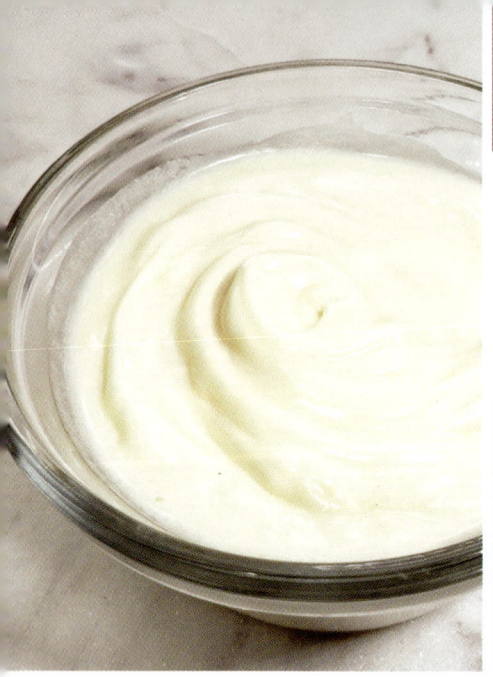

CARNIVORE MAYONNAISE

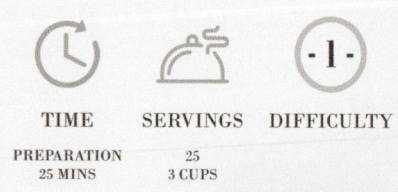

TIME
PREPARATION
25 MINS

SERVINGS
25
3 CUPS

DIFFICULTY
-1-

- PER SERVING -
42 CALORIES
PROTEIN: 1G
CARBS: 0G
FATS: 4G

INGREDIENTS

½ Cup of Room Temperature Duck Fat
½ Cup of Egg Whites
2 Tsp of Redmond Real Salt
1 Tbsp of White Vinegar
1 Whole Large Egg

STEPS

- 1 - Mix all ingredients together in a blender or food processor.

- 2 - Blend for 3 minutes or until everything has been fully incorporated into each other.

- 3 - Refrigerate for 2 hours before using it.

   Note If duck fat is melted, refrigerating will take longer.

SPICY MAYONNAISE

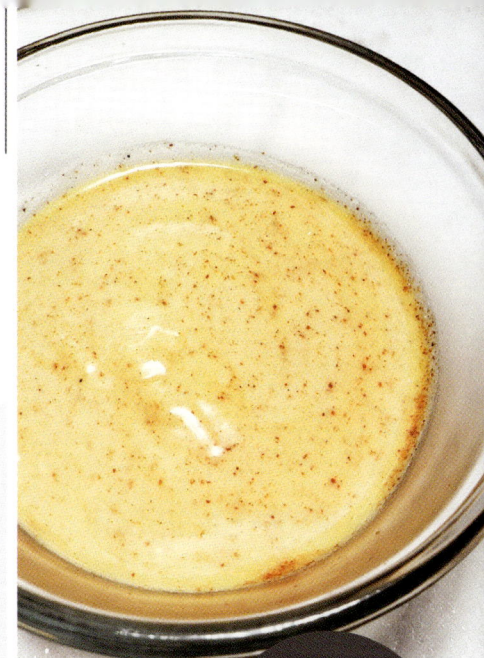

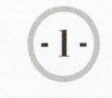 

DIFFICULTY -1-   **SERVINGS** 25   **TIME** PREPARATION 25 MINS

PER SERVING
42 CALORIES
PROTEIN: 1G
CARBS: 0G
FATS: 4G

INGREDIENTS

½ Cup of Room Temperature Duck Fat
½ Cup of Egg Whites
2 Tbsp of Sugar Free Hot Sauce
2 Tsp of Redmond Real Salt
1 Tbsp of White Vinegar
1 Whole Large Egg

STEPS

- 1 - Add all ingredients to a food processor or blender.

- 2 - Mix together thoroughly by blending for 3-5 minutes.

- 3 - Refrigerate for 2 hours before using.

The Ultimate Carnivore Cookbook / 111
www.bioptimizedketo.com

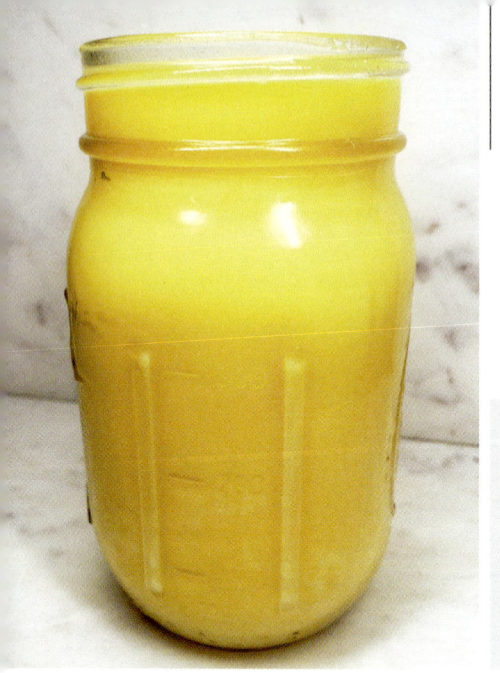

GARLIC GHEE

TIME
PREPARATION
15 MINS
COOKING
45 MINS

SERVINGS
30

DIFFICULTY
-1-

-PER SERVING-
78 CALORIES
PROTEIN: 0G
CARBS: 0G
FATS: 9G

INGREDIENTS

10 Oz of Ghee
8 Cloves of Peeled Garlic

STEPS

- 1 -   Add ghee and garlic cloves to a pot.

- 2 -   Heat the pot to medium heat and stir frequently.

- 3 -   Poach the garlic cloves in the ghee for 35 minutes.

- 4 -   Remove the garlic cloves from the pot and pour the ghee into a Mason jar through a strainer.

Note Can be stored safely out of a refrigerator for 3 months or 9 months inside the refrigerator.

GARLIC HOLLANDAISE SAUCE

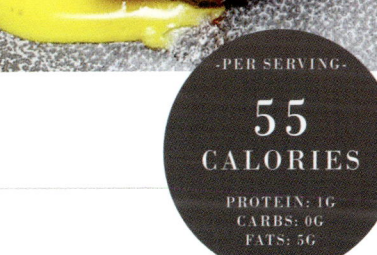

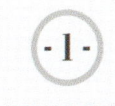  

DIFFICULTY: 1
SERVINGS: 4
TIME: PREPARATION 20 MINS

PER SERVING
55 CALORIES
PROTEIN: 1G
CARBS: 0G
FATS: 5G

INGREDIENTS

2½ Tbsp of Garlic Ghee* (see recipe)
2 Large Egg Yolks

STEPS

- 1 - Melt the Ghee and set to the side.
- 2 - Crack the eggs and separate the egg whites and yolks from each other, placing the yolks into a mixing bowl.
- 3 - Whisk the yolks until smooth.
- 4 - Slowly add the ghee to the egg yolks in small increments while continuing to whisk vigorously.

    Note This is to avoid the ghee from cooking the yolks.

- 5 - Keep whisking until it thickens.
- 6 - Serve immediately or refrigerate for later use.

The Ultimate Carnivore Cookbook
www.bioptimizedketo.com

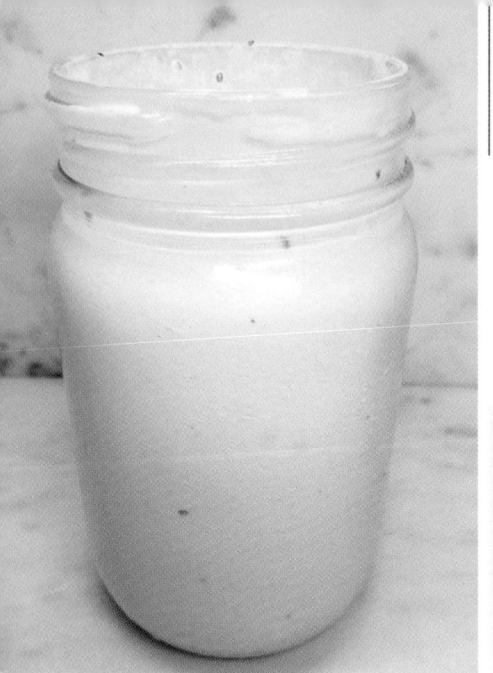

RANCH DRESSING

  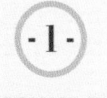

TIME   SERVINGS   DIFFICULTY

PREPARATION 15 MINS   25

-PER SERVING-

34 CALORIES

PROTEIN: 0G
CARBS: 0G
FATS: 3G

INGREDIENTS

½ Cup of Carnivore Mayo* (see recipe)
½ Cup of Sour Cream or Greek Yogurt
½ Cup of Heavy Cream
1 Tsp of White Vinegar
½ Tsp of Redmond Real Salt
½ Tsp of Fresh Cracked Pepper

STEPS

- 1 - Add all ingredients to a food processor or blender and pulse until mixed together.

- 2 - Can be used immediately after making or refrigerated for later use.

BEEF BONE BROTH

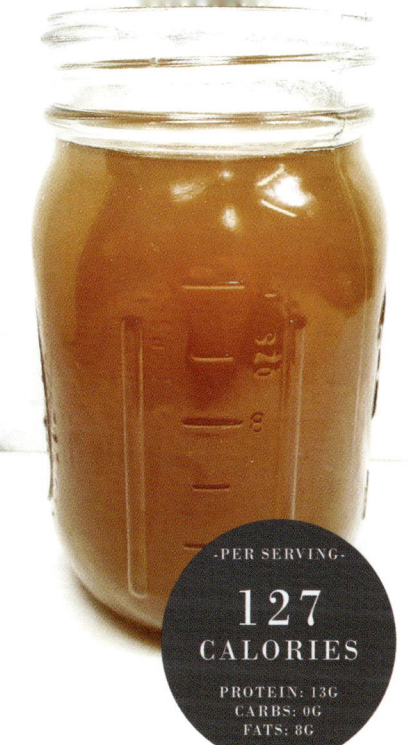

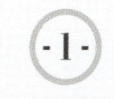		
DIFFICULTY	SERVINGS	TIME
	8	PREPARATION 10 MINS
		COOKING 24-36 HOURS

PER SERVING
127 CALORIES
PROTEIN: 13G
CARBS: 0G
FATS: 8G

INGREDIENTS

2 Pounds of Beef Bones
1½ Tsp of Redmond Real Salt

1 Tsp of White Vinegar
½ Gallon of Filtered Water

STEPS

- 1 - In a slow cooker or crockpot, add the beef bones.

- 2 - Pour in the water until the bones are almost completely submerged.

- 3 - Add the salt and vinegar.

- 4 - Turn the slow cooker on to low heat and cook for 24 to 36 hours.

- 5 - After cooking, strain out the bones and other solids and store in Mason jars.

    Note Can be refrigerated for 5 days or frozen for up to 5 months.

The Ultimate Carnivore Cookbook /
www.bioptimizedketo.com

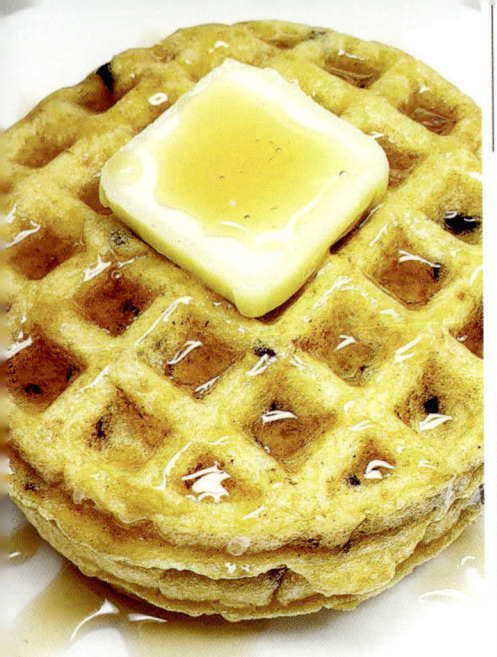

CARNIVORE-ISH CHOCOLATE CHIP WAFFLES

TIME
PREPARATION 25 MINS
COOKING 25 MINS

SERVINGS 4

DIFFICULTY -1-

-PER SERVING-
445 CALORIES
PROTEIN: 41G
CARBS: 2G
FATS: 31G

INGREDIENTS

2 Cups of Pork Panko by Bacon's Heir
2 Large Eggs
2½ Tbsp of Egg Whites
1 Tbsp of Organic Cacao Nibs
½ Tsp of SweetLeaf Stevia Vanilla Créme Sweetener
Sugar-Free Maple Syrup and Butter for Topping

STEPS

- 1 -   Mix ingredients all together thoroughly in a bowl.

- 2 -   Scoop batter into a waffle iron and cook.

- 3 -   Top with butter and sugar free maple syrup.

CARNIVORE-ISH FRENCH TOAST STICKS

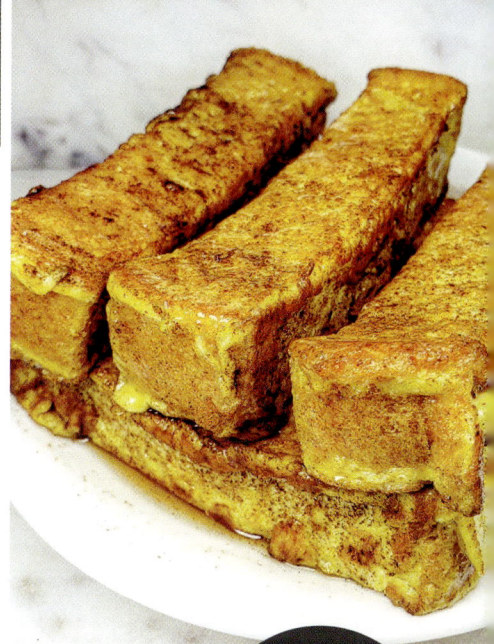

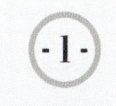
DIFFICULTY

SERVINGS
4

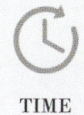
TIME
PREPARATION
25 MINS
COOKING
20 MINS

-PER SERVING-
494 CALORIES
PROTEIN: 39G
CARBS: 2G
FATS: 36G

INGREDIENTS

3 Slices of Carnivore Bread* (see recipe)
2 Large Eggs
2 Tsp of Butter
¼ Cup of Heavy Cream (Optional)
1½ Tbsp of Cinnamon
Sugar-Free Maple Syrup for Topping/Dipping

STEPS

- 1 -   Cut thick slices off of a loaf of Carnivore Bread.

- 2 -   Cut those slices into strips.

- 3 -   In a bowl, crack and scramble the eggs and add in the heavy cream.

- 4 -   Mix together.

The Ultimate Carnivore Cookbook / 117
www.bioptimizedketo.com

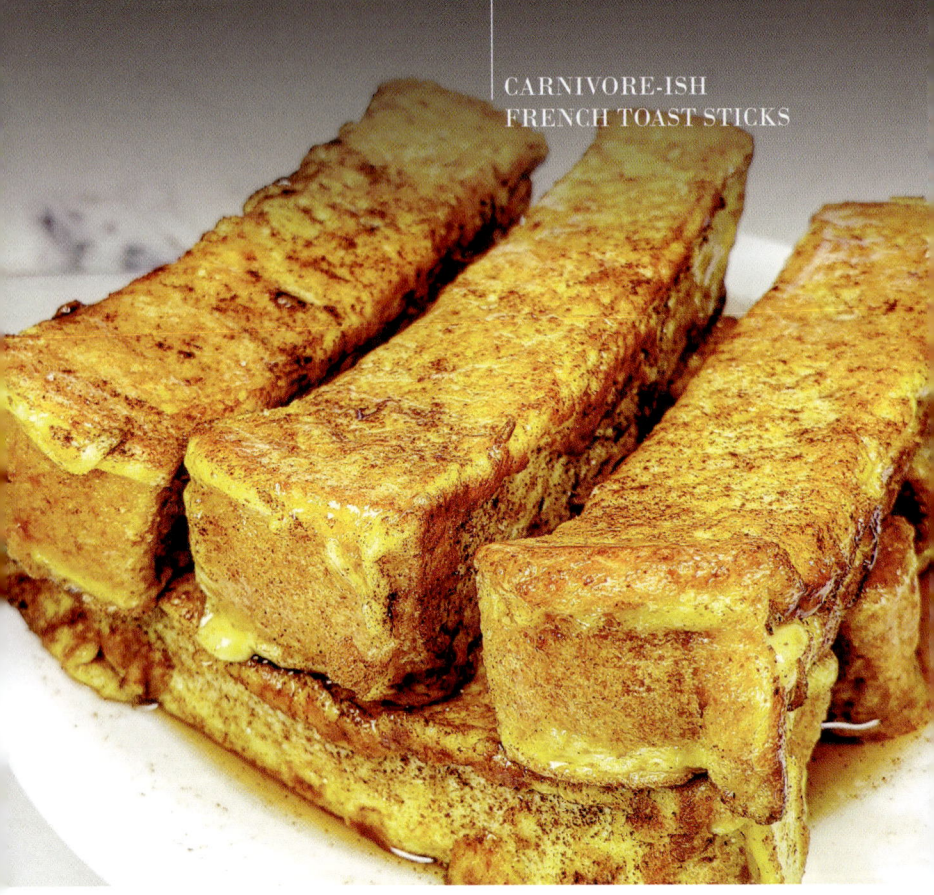

CARNIVORE-ISH FRENCH TOAST STICKS

STEPS

- 5 - Submerge the bread strips into the bowl 3 at a time and allow them to soak up the mixture.

- 6 - Heat a nonstick pan to medium heat with the butter.

- 7 - Move the bread strips from the bowl directly into the pan.

- 8 - Fry in the pan until golden brown and repeat for all 4 sides of the sticks.

- 9 - Remove from the pan and sprinkle the cinnamon on top.

- 10 - Plate and serve with sugar-free maple syrup.

CARNIVORE TAFFY

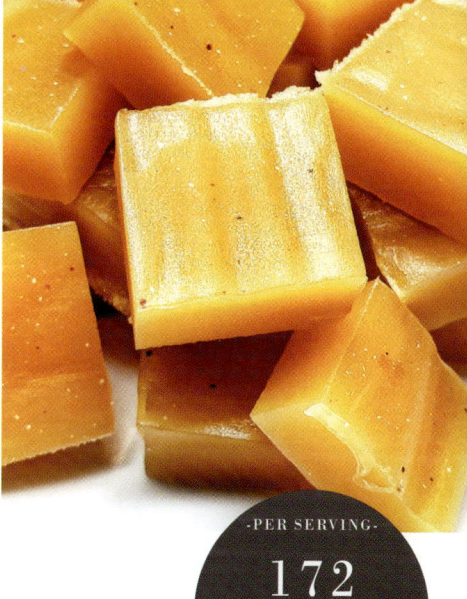

  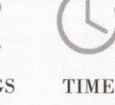

DIFFICULTY 1
SERVINGS 30
TIME COOKING 35 MINS

PER SERVING
172 CALORIES
PROTEIN: 16G
CARBS: 0G
FATS: 12G

INGREDIENTS

480 Grams of Collagen Peptides
40 Grams of Gelatin
2 Cups of Unsalted Butter
2 Cups of Filtered Water
1½ Tsp of Redmond Real Salt
10 Drops of Liquid Stevia or Monk Fruit

STEPS

- 1 -   In a large pot, add butter, salt and water.

- 2 -   Heat to a medium heat and stir together.

- 3 -   Line a deep baking dish with parchment paper.

- 4 -   Once it's heated and mixed completely add the gelatin and mix thoroughly.

The Ultimate Carnivore Cookbook / 119
www.bioptimizedketo.com

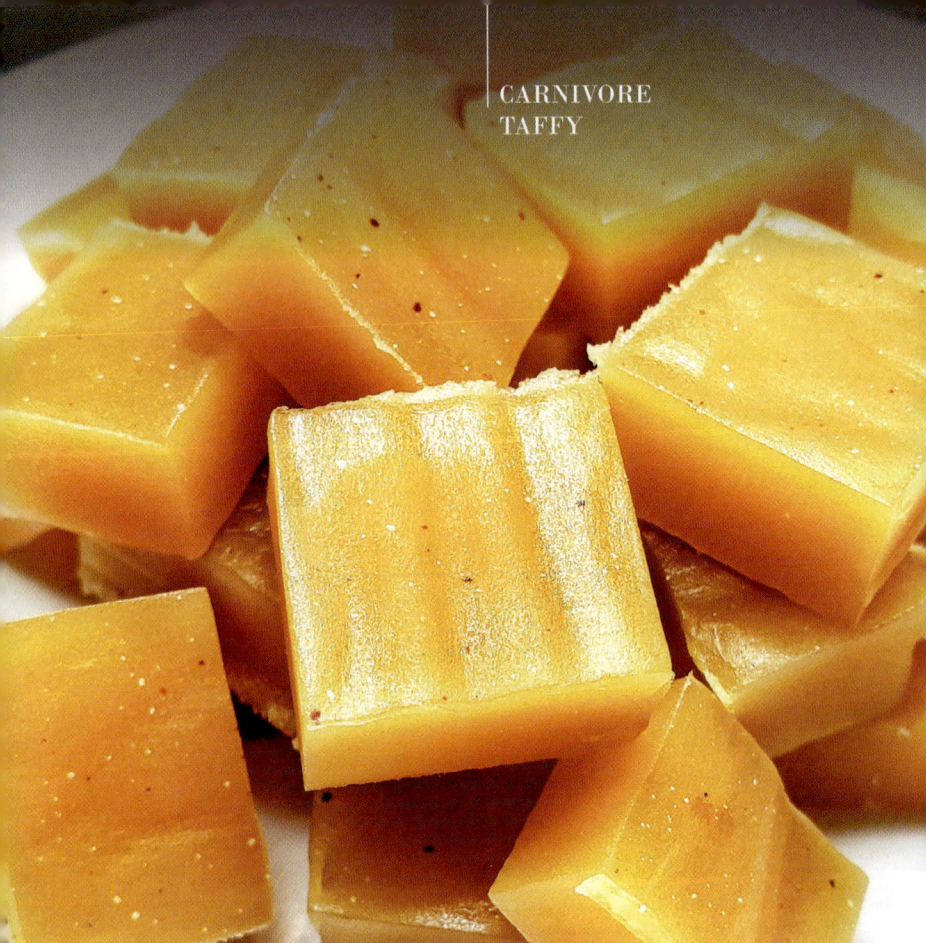

CARNIVORE TAFFY

STEPS

- 5 - In portions slowly add the collagen peptides while mixing with an immersion blender.

- 6 - Continue mixing with the immersion blender while adding all of the collagen.

- 7 - Blend until there are no lumps of powders and everything looks smooth.

- 8 - After blending, pour into the lined baking dish and refrigerate overnight.

CARNIVORE-ISH CINNAMON ROLL

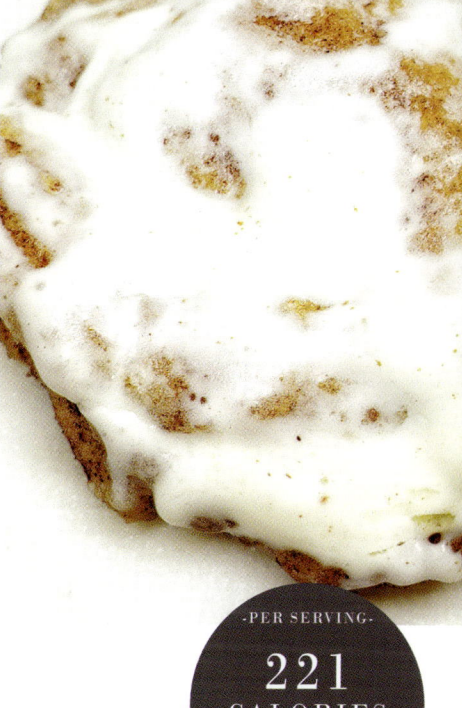

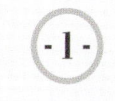  

DIFFICULTY: 1
SERVINGS: 6
TIME: PREPARATION 35 MINS / COOKING 25 MINS

·PER SERVING·
221 CALORIES
PROTEIN: 16G
CARBS: 3G
FATS: 16G

INGREDIENTS

100 Grams of Vanilla Protein Powder
14 Tsp of Softened Butter
10 Drops of Sweetleaf Vanilla Créme Liquid Stevia
5 Tsp of Ground Cinnamon
⅓ Cup of Cream Cheese
1 Tbsp of Heavy Cream
½ Cup of Water
2 Large Eggs

STEPS

- 1 - Mix protein powder and 2 tsp of cinnamon together in a bowl.

- 2 - Add 8 tsp of butter in small pieces into the bowl and mix thoroughly.

- 3 - Add the eggs and then mix again.

- 4 - Slowly add the water and mix until its fully incorporated into the dough.

The Ultimate Carnivore Cookbook / 121
www.bioptimizedketo.com

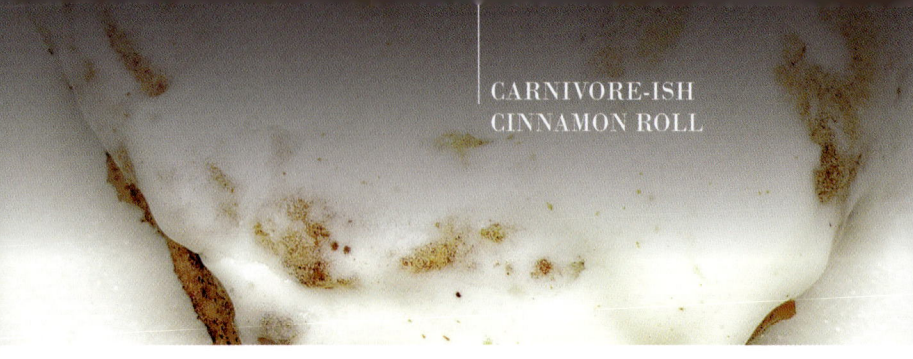

CARNIVORE-ISH CINNAMON ROLL

STEPS

- 5 - Scoop the dough onto a large piece of parchment and roll between another piece of parchment until the dough is 1-inch thick rectangle.

- 6 - Preheat the oven to 350°F.

- 7 - Create the filling by mixing 3 tsp of butter and 3 tsp of cinnamon to a small bowl.

- 8 - Mix thoroughly with a fork.

- 9 - Spread the filling evenly over the dough.

- 10 - Roll the dough and cut into 6 to 8 segments.

- 11 - Line a baking dish with parchment paper and place each roll into the pan on the flat side.

- 12 - Place into the oven and bake for 25 minutes.

- 13 - While the rolls bake, make the icing by adding 3 tsp of butter, ⅓ cup of cream cheese, 1 tbsp of heavy cream and 10 drops of the Liquid Stevia.

- 14 - Mix thoroughly and set to the side until the Cinnamon Rolls are finished baking.

- 15 - After removing the Cinnamon Rolls from the oven, cover in the Icing while they are still hot.

- 16 - Serve and enjoy.

CARNIVORE-ISH BROWNIE

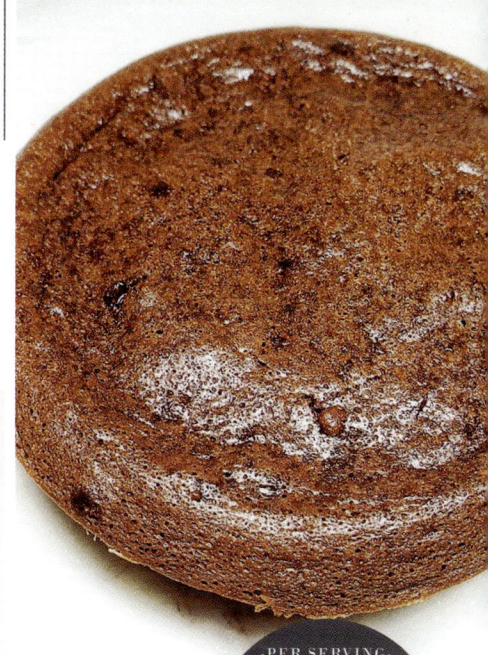

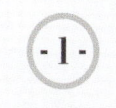
DIFFICULTY -1-

SERVINGS 4

TIME
PREPARATION 25 MINS
COOKING 30 MINS

-PER SERVING-
148 CALORIES
PROTEIN: 17G
CARBS: 1G
FATS: 8G

INGREDIENTS

2 Scoops of Equip Foods Chocolate Protein Powder
15 Grams of Unflavored Collagen Peptides
6 Tsp of Butter
2 Large Eggs
1 Tsp of Redmond Real Salt
10 Drops of Lakanto Chocolate flavored Liquid Monk Fruit Drops

STEPS

- 1 -   Preheat the oven to 350°F.

- 2 -   Mix all dry ingredients together in a bowl.

- 3 -   Melt the butter and then add the eggs, mixing together thoroughly.

  Note Make sure the butter cools off before adding the eggs or it will cook the eggs.

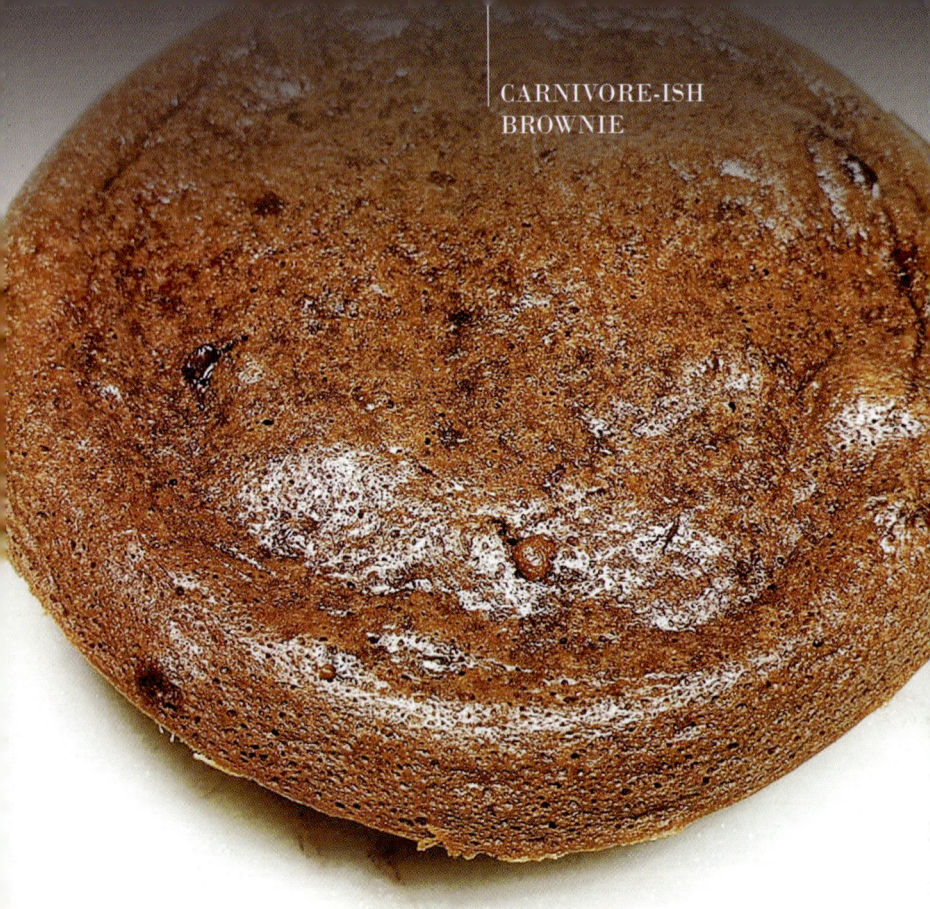

CARNIVORE-ISH BROWNIE

STEPS

- 4 - Add the wet ingredients to the dry ingredients slowly and mix together.

   Note The mixture may get tough to mix. If it gets too hard, add a tbsp of filtered water.

- 5 - After mixing, scoop into a muffin top baking pan.

- 6 - Place the pan into the oven and bake for 30 minutes.

- 7 - Remove from the oven and enjoy.

FIX THE STRESS

OPTIMAL LEVELS OF THIS ALL-NATURAL NUTRIENT HELPS ANXIETY, RELAXATION AND STRESS-RELIEF

- Reduce your stress levels and feel relaxed and at peace
- Sleep faster and deeper
- Boost your immune system
- Maintain normal heart rhythm
- Lowering cortisol levels
- Build strong bones

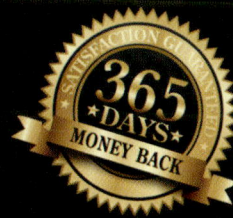

For more information visit **www.bioptimizers.com**

Keep out of reach of children. As with any product, discontinue immediately if adverse effects occur.
Please consult a physician before beginning any new supplement, diet, training program, or if you are undergoing treatment of a medical condition.

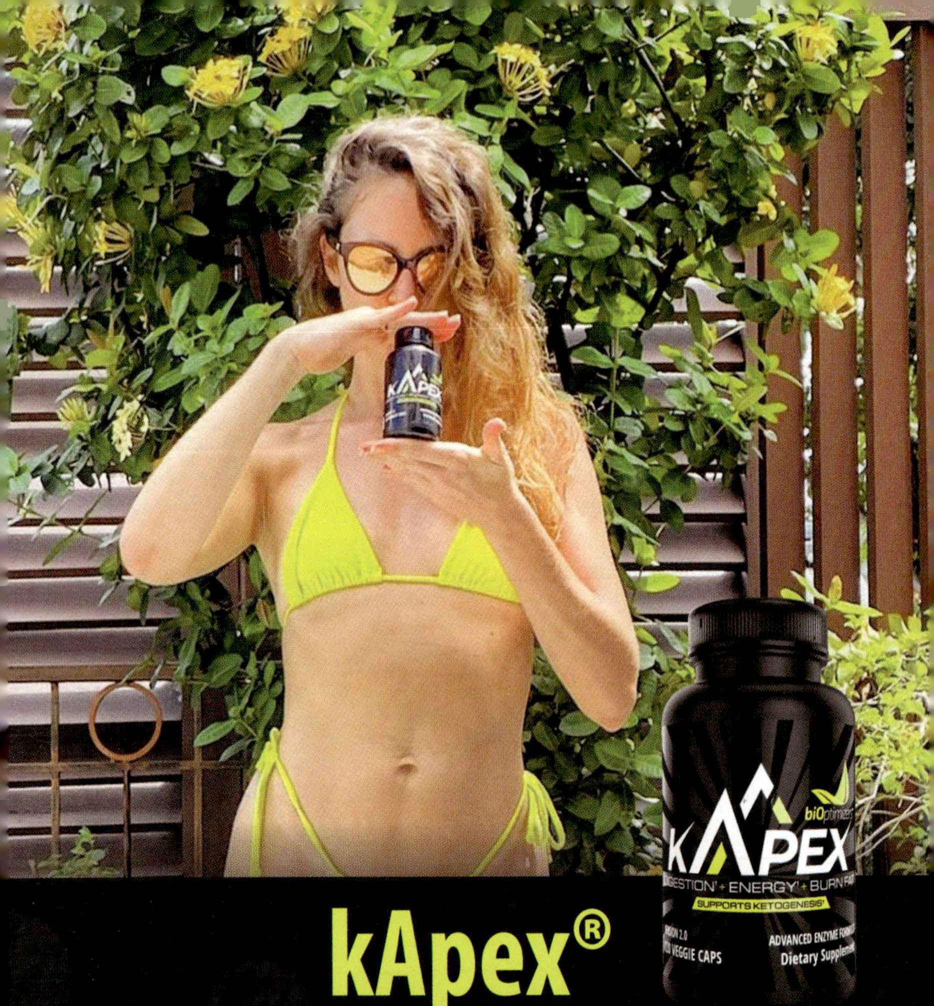

kApex®

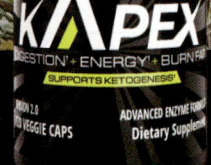

IMPROVE KETO, LOW-CARB, PALEO DIGESTION, AND INCREASE ENERGY

- Boosts AMPK in muscles by 52% and fat cells by 300%
- Ups ATP in your liver by 22% (a key part of energy)
- Amps adiponectin by up to 248%
- Lifts glut4 up to 488%—which is the insulin-regulated glucose transporter.
- Helps lower inflammation and more ...

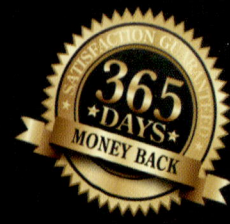

For more information visit **www.bioptimizers.com**

Keep out of reach of children. As with any product, discontinue immediately if adverse effects occur. Please consult a physician before beginning any new supplement, diet, training program, or if you are undergoing treatment of a medical condition.